12-26-62

12-26-62

FOLKLORE and ODYSSEYS of FOOD and MEDICINAL PLANTS

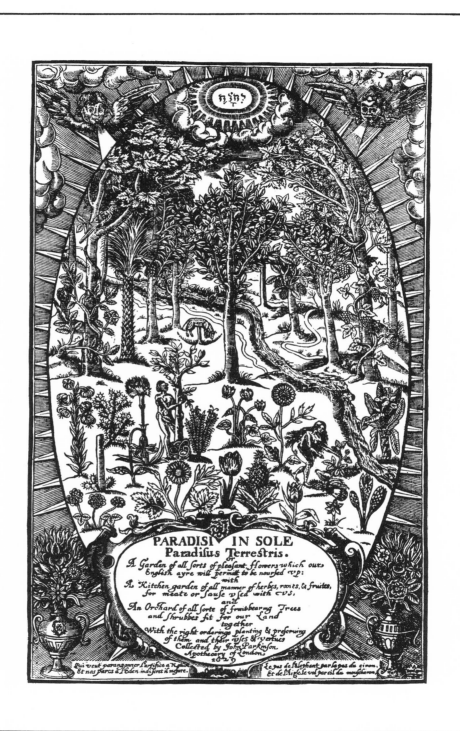

Title Page, from John Parkinson's PARADISI IN SOLE, *London, 1629.*

FOLKLORE and ODYSSEYS

OF

FOOD and MEDICINAL PLANTS

By

ERNST and JOHANNA LEHNER

TUDOR PUBLISHING COMPANY
New York, N.Y.

To Our Dear Friend Ruth Goldberg

CONTENTS

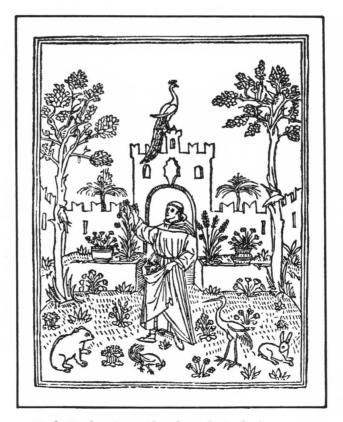

Herb Garden, from Cherubino da Spaloti's FIOR DE VIRTU, *Venice, 1490.*

INTRODUCTION

EREALS AND FRUITS, salads and vegetables, beverages and stimulants are the pillars of our daily diet. When we sit down to breakfast, lunch or dinner, take a snack or a bracer in between meals, we never fully realize that we are so well supplied with food only because generation after generation of human beings have used themselves as guinea pigs to find out by trial and error which of all the many thousands of plants around the globe were edible. We forget that at some time, somewhere, everything that covers the earth has been tried for edibility by humans, out of curiosity or necessity, many times with pleasure and delight, sometimes with catastrophic results. And the sum-total of all this pioneer work of bygone generations is the filling of our present-day kitchen shelves, vegetable bins, refrigerators, pantries, cellars and medicine cabinets. We also do not realize that the greater number of our grains, vegetables, herbs, fruits, condiments and stimulants are not native to wherever we are but originated hundreds, sometimes thousands, of years ago on other continents. It took many voyages, expeditions, intrigues and wars, much toil and sweat to bring to our doorsteps and backyards those plants which we take as a matter of course. For the discovery of many of these plants, their travels from one continent to another, knowledge of their properties and cultivation, their abundant presence today in our fields and gardens, our primary thanks are due the scholars of antiquity such as the Greek historian Herodotus (484-425 B.C.), whose explorations took him to northern Africa, Egypt, Assyria, and Persia; the ancient conquerors such as Alexander the Great, King of Macedon (356-323 B.C.), whose military thrusts led him into Persia and India; the empire builders such as Harun-al-Rashid, Caliph of Bagdad (766-809 A.D.), whose influential contacts reached from the Tang dynasty emperors of the East to the court of Charlemagne, King of the Franks and Emperor of the West; the medieval merchant princes such as the Venetian Marco Polo (1254-1324), whose extensive travels brought him to Kublai Khan's Mongolia and Cathay (China); the Roman legions and the Mohammedan Saracens; the Christian crusaders and the Turkish Mameluks; the Spanish *conquistadores* and the mariners and explorers of many lands. All took along the seeds of their native plants wherever they went and, in return, brought home for transplantation whatever they found. When the first white settlers arrived in North America, they found in the beginning a dull fare of maize, beans, squash, sweet potatoes, berries, nuts, maple syrup, and odds and ends. Considerable time elapsed before they were able to import seeds and cuttings and to cultivate on American soil all the commonplace cereals, vegetables, fruits and herbs on our tables today. As time progressed more new settlers arrived and newer and vastly different species of plants were introduced. From western Asia and Europe came the cereal grains, the sugar beet, and the carrot. From the Orient came rice. From South and Latin America, the tomato made its bow. Still later, the cabbage, the lettuce, and the turnip made their auspicious debuts. Alcoholic spirit beverages were brought in from every country of the globe along with a wide variety of the herbs and fruits from which they were brewed.

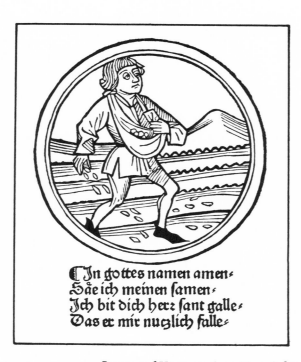 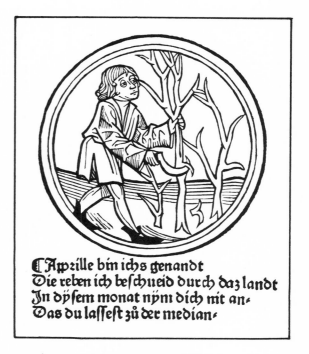

Sower and Vintager, from Hans Schönsperger's AUGSBURGER KALENDER, *1487.*

THE CEREALS

THE STORY OF AGRICULTURE

NTOLD MILLENNIA AGO the cave man consumed as vegetable food the leaves, stalks, roots, fruit, nuts and seed gathered by the women and children of his tribe in the jungles and forests surrounding his habitat. He was forced to drift north and south with the seasons in pursuit of his food. One day he discovered that the seed dropped by accident near his cave grew into new seed-producing plants. It gave him the idea of planting seeds purposely near his dwelling place and, finally, of clearing a patch of ground, preparing it by loosening the sod with a crooked stick, (the first hoe), and seeding it. Thus man changed from a nomadic *poacher* roaming for food, to a settled *farmer*, waiting for his next harvest. With the growth of the tribe, more and more cleared acreage became necessary to meet the rising demand for food, and more manpower was needed to prepare and till the fields. Ultimately, man decided that the established law of the jungle, to kill all his enemies (the members of other tribes) immediately after they were taken prisoner on his hunting forays, was wasteful. He brought them home and put them to work on his fields — the first forced-labor slaves in human history. They call for still more intensive food production for the rising population of these settlements led to the idea of harnessing domesticated animals to the *hoe*. Thus the *plow* became the new tool of agriculture. Agriculture is the scientific term for the art of cultivating the soil. The word is

THE STORY OF AGRICULTURE

derived from the Latin *ager* — field, and *cultura* — tilling. The name cereals is derived from the Latin *cerealis* — pertaining to Ceres, the Roman goddess of vegetation. It refers to all food-grain bearing grasses, as barley, buckwheat, maize or Indian corn, millet, oats, rice, rye, wheat, etc. The cereals originated in Central Asia and the Far East, with the exception of Indian corn,

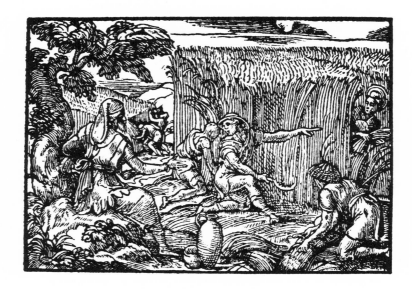

Ruth and Boaz, from Derendel's THE WOLL BIBLE, *Lyons, 1553.*

THE STORY OF AGRICULTURE

native to South America. They have been cultivated since prehistoric times, and their distribution became world-wide as civilization advanced. The practice of agriculture was the necessary antecedent to a higher form of cultural development, and wherever great states and empires were founded, cereals were grown as staple foods. The cultures of antiquity were all built

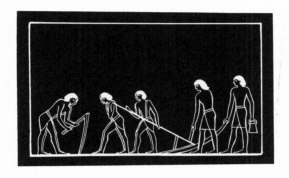

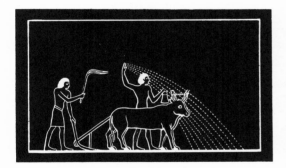
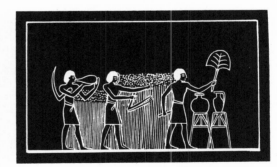

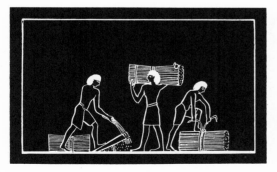
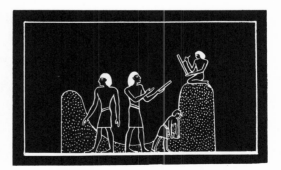

Farming in Ancient Egypt, from an antique wall painting.

THE STORY OF AGRICULTURE

around the agricultural centers of grain-growing peoples: the Chinese, Indians, Koreans and Japanese in Asia; the Sumerians, Babylonians, Assyrians, Hittites, Phoenicians, Israelites and Syrians in the Near East; the Egyptians, Lydians, Nubians and Carthaginians in Africa; the Cretans, Greeks, Etruscans and Romans in Europe; the Incas, Mayas and Aztecs in South and

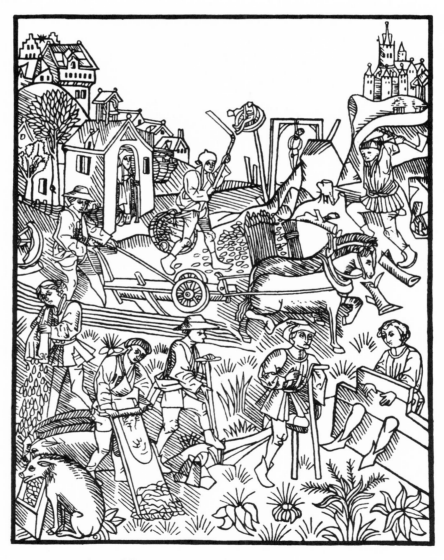

Farming in the Middle Ages, from WIRKUNG DER PLANETEN, *Germany, 1470.*

THE STORY OF AGRICULTURE

Central America. When we look at the farming methods and implements in the 15th, 16th and 17th centuries, we marvel at the thought that for nearly 7000 years of agricultural development the methods and tools of the toilers in the fields did not change very much. In our century of industrialization we saw the rise of the mechanical behemoths of modern farming machinery,

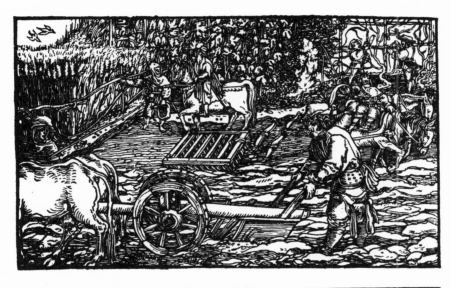

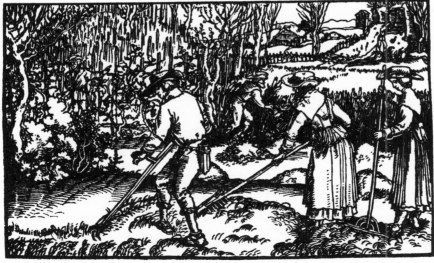

German Agriculture, from Petrarca's TROSTSPIEGEL, *Augsburg, 1532.*

THE STORY OF AGRICULTURE

the reaper and the cotton gin, which not only boomed the agrarian economy of western nations but enhanced the process of industrialization and became a leading factor in the eventual establishment of the western nations as great world markets. Newer developments in the field of chemistry led to still further uses for the products of agriculture. Thus today we find need

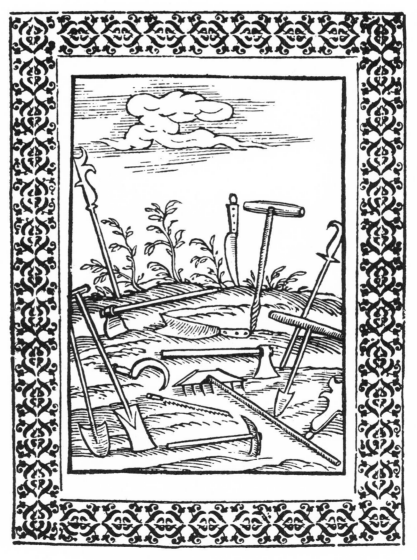

Gardening Tools, from Pusato's GIARDINO DI AGRICULTURA, *Venice, 1593.*

THE STORY OF AGRICULTURE

for plants and herbs not only as sources of food, clothing and medicine, but for such hundreds of newly developed industrial needs as stagger the imagination. However, we have to realize, that to this very day in large parts of South America, Africa, and the Far East the agricultural methods and the farming tools are still nearly the same as in Biblical times.

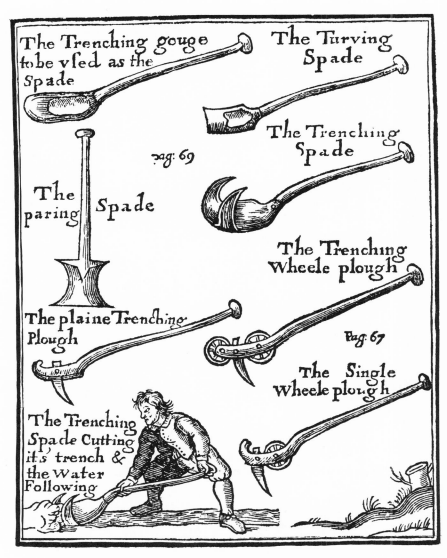

Farming Tools, from Blith's THE ENGLISH IMPROVER IMPROVED, *London, 1652.*

THE STORY OF BARLEY

Barley (*Hordeum vulgare*) is a cereal grass of unknown origin, cultivated since prehistoric times in many parts of the world. It seems to be one of the first grains grown by man as a staple food. Barley may have once been native to Asia, from which nearly all of our cereals come, but grains of it have been found in such diverse places as Egyptian remains from the Pre-Dynastic period (5000 B.C.), Babylonian tombs (300 B.C.), Bronze Age pile-dwellings of the Hallstatt period (1500 B.C.), and in the Alpine lakes of Austria and Switzerland. The Egyptians, Sumerians, Babylonians and Assyrians knew all about the use of barley for alcoholic beverages, and the oldest known recipe for *barley-wine* was found in a cruciform inscription on a Babylonian library brick (2800 B.C.). Barley is frequently mentioned in the Books of Moses, and the ancient Greeks trained their athletes on barley-mush because it was considered the mildest of all cereals. Barley was well known in ancient India and was dedicated to Indra who was called *He who ripens barley*. Hindus use its grains in their religious celebrations, at weddings, childbirths, funerals and other rites. In ancient China, the seed-rich, heavy-bearded barley was a symbol of male potency. Today the use of barley in bread is indicative of poverty and the greatest part of the world's crop is consumed in the form of malted beverages.

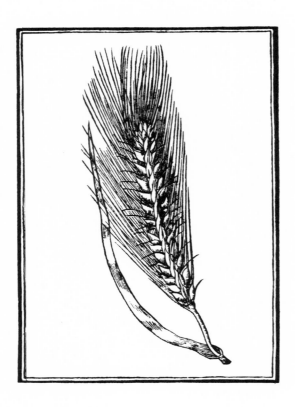

Barley, from Mattioli's COMMENTAIRES, *Lyons, 1579.*

THE STORY OF BUCKWHEAT

Buckwheat (*Fagopyrum esculentum*), a grain cereal native to Tatary, was widely cultivated in Central Asia and the Near East. Crusaders who fought the Saracens in the Holy Land in the 12th century brought the seed of buckwheat back to Europe, and in France it is still called *blés sarrasin* — Saracen corn. Its English name is derived from the Anglo-Saxon *boc* — beech, because its grain has a triangular shape resembling that of a beechnut. Buckwheat is one of the staple grains of the Far East; the Japanese, for example, are great consumers of buckwheat noodles, called *Soba.* Japanese goldsmiths have long used buckwheat dough to collect the gold dust in their shops, and the grain is therefore considered a potent charm for collecting riches. Every Japanese family eats buckwheat noodles on New Year's Eve in order to acquire the luck for amassing money in the coming year; and every household prepares and serves *soba* on all festive occasions. When a Japanese moves to a new house, he gives a present of *soba* to all his neighbors; to the neighbors on each side, and to the three across the road from his new home. This expresses his wish for their good fortune and for a long lasting friendship. Today buckwheat is cultivated throughout Asia, Europe and the North American continent, with buckwheat griddle cakes being widely enjoyed in the United States.

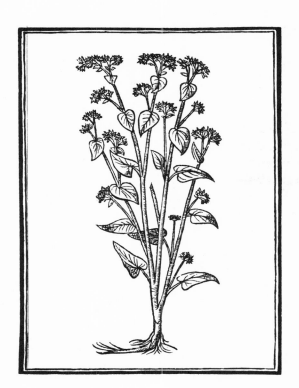

Buckwheat, from Mattioli's COMMENTAIRES, *Lyons, 1579.*

THE STORY OF MAIZE

Cinteotl, the Maize God of the Mayan Indians.

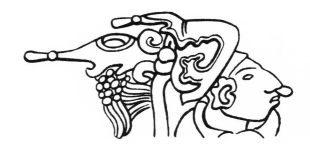

The cultivation of maize or Indian corn *(Zea mays)*, a plant native to the Americas, ante-dates Christopher Columbus' discovery of the New World by nearly 3,000 years. The Aztecs, Mayas, Incas and other Indian tribes were all descendents of maize-growing agricultural peoples who inhabited the middle Americas in early antiquity. Their gods were personifications of nature. Maize, a life-giving god itself, was treated with the greatest veneration. Even loose kernels on the ground were never stepped upon, but picked up carefully since they were regarded as part of the deity. In all of the Americas, maize-growing tribes had their corn-gods,

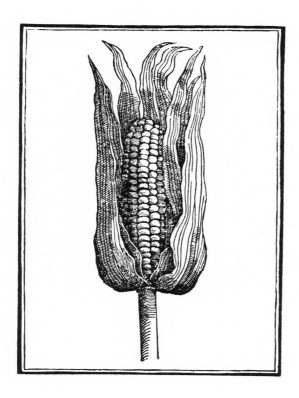

Maize, from Oviedo y Valdés' HISTORIA NATURAL, Seville, 1535.

THE STORY OF MAIZE

corn-mothers or corn-maidens, deities of maize, revered by special corn-sowing dances, rain ceremonies, prayer-rites for the sprouting seed, and festivals of thanks at harvest time. All of these tribes, from South America to our eastern seaboard, had scores of tales about how maize came to their lands. According to a legend of the Narraganset Indians, for example, one day in very early history, a crow came from the southwest to their hunting grounds bearing a kernel of corn in one ear, and, in the other, a bean. This is how their vegetable crops originated. From that time on, the legend proceeds, crows feasting in their corn and bean fields were never molested, for they were entitled to partake of the harvest which one of their ancestors had made possible. In 1496 Columbus brought the first sample of maize from the Caribbean to Spain and, in the following century, maize was planted in Europe from the Atlantic to the Ural Mountains. It became an important crop in every European country, one of the agricultural gifts of the New World to the Old. In the first half of the 16th century, European herbalists nearly succeeded in depriving the New World of the distinction that maize had originated in the Americas. These herbalists named the new plant *Welsh corn, Asiatic corn* or *Turkish corn* because they believed that the plant had been brought by the Turks from Asia. It was an understandable mistake, because it was at this time that the Turks invaded Europe, and brought scores of new items never seen before in the west. Everything unusual at this time was labeled *"Turkish."* It took the Spanish botanists over half a century to convince their European fellow herbalists

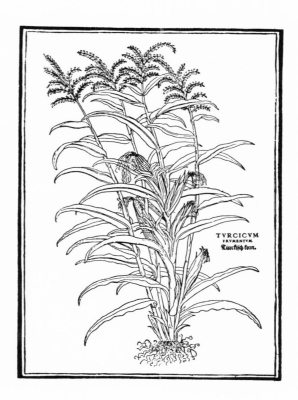

Turkish Corn, from Fuchs' DE HISTORIA STIRPIUM, *Basle, 1542.*

THE STORY OF MAIZE

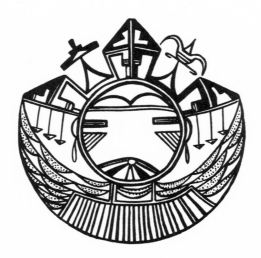

Shalako Mana, the Corn Mist Maiden of the Hopi Indians.

that Columbus had brought the plant from the New World, and that it should rightly be labeled *Maize*, or *India corn*. Our native American bird, the *Turkey*, misnamed in Europe at the same time for the same reason, was not so lucky and has consequently continued to bear that wrong name ever since. Even today, few Americans realize why this indigenous fowl bears the name of a Near Eastern nation. Today, in addition to corn-on-the-cob being a culinary favorite, corn has become a major ingredient in breakfast cereals and found numerous uses in cooking and baking. Apart from its value as a food, one of its most important uses is in the form of fermented grain from which a wide variety of alcoholic spirit beverages are produced. Popcorn, a special type of Indian corn, has found widespread popularity as a confection and an appetizing snack. Cornstarch has become an important household item in both cooking and laundering. Cornbread has been a long-time supplement on the American dinner table.

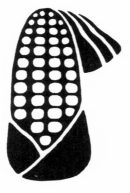

Aztec Maize Symbol of Fertility, Veracruz.

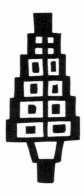

Maize Symbol of the Pueblo Indians.

THE STORY OF MILLET

Millet *(Panicum miliaceum)* is a cereal grass, native to the East Indies, where it has been cultivated since time immemorial. Its pearly seeds are the smallest of all cereal grains. Millet was known in ancient Babylonia and Assyria, and the Greek historian, Herodotus, brought the knowledge of it back from his extensive journeys into the Near East in the 5th Century B.C. Cultivation of millet was propagated all over Africa and Europe, and today it is extensively grown not only in India, Ceylon, and other countries in the Far and Near East; but also in east and central Africa, and in southern Europe. In America it is cultivated mostly for use as a cattle and poultry feed.

Millet, from Mattioli's COMMENTAIRES, *Lyons, 1579.*

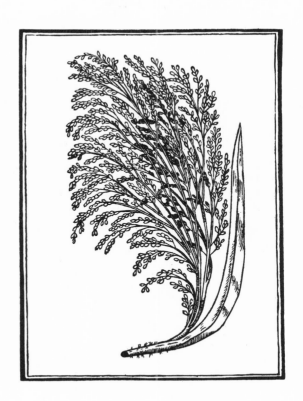

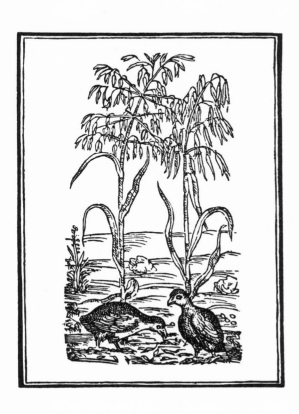

THE STORY OF OATS

The common oat *(Avena sativa)* was, like its main consumer, the horse, native to Tatary in Central Asia. About 2000 B.C., when the domesticated horse was brought from Asia to Arabia and Egypt, the cultivation of oats went along as the necessary staple for these newly-acquired animals. Even in ancient Greece and Rome, the planting of oats accompanied the introduction of the horse. This same pattern persisted in the course of the Roman conquests of Europe and the British Isles. Oats accordingly became a major crop for human consumption in Norway, Sweden, Ireland and Scotland, especially since they acclimatized themselves well to the colder regions of the north.

Oats, from Mattioli's COMMENTARII, *Venice, 1560.*

THE STORY OF RICE

The common rice *(Oryza sativa)* is not only one of the oldest, but also the most extensively cultivated of all grain cereals. It is the staple food for nearly half of the world's population: from China, Korea, Japan and the Philippines, to India, Burma, Siam, Bali, Malaya, and all the islands from Formosa to Madagascar. It is the central food of the Far East where, in fact, meat, fish, fowl, vegetables and condiments are considered only garnishes for the main dish of rice. According to Chinese tradition, the legendary Emperor Shun-Nung (2800-2700 B.C.) taught the Chinese people the art of cultivating rice. For over 4500 years — as long as the "Kingdom of the Middle" (Imperial China) existed — every 5th of February, the day of Li-Chun, the Emperor of China and his princes, ministers, governors and mandarins went to selected rice fields near their palaces and got behind the plough to start the tilling season. The Emperor would furrow 3 rows, the princes 6, the court ministers 9, the governors 12 and the mandarins 15. The people would take pieces of the newly upturned earth from these fields and scatter the dust over their own rice paddies to assure a bountiful crop in the coming year. Rice is so highly regarded by the Chinese that their equivalent to our daily greeting, *How do you do?* is *Have you eaten your rice today?*. Rice is a symbol of fertility and as such was originally used in China to pelt newlywed couples in order to bring them good luck and assure them of many children. The upsetting of a rice bowl on the table or elsewhere is a very unlucky omen, and to take a

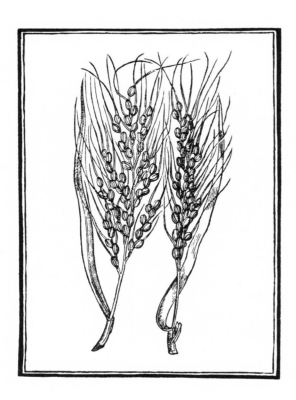

Rice, from Mattioli's COMMENTAIRES, *Lyons, 1579.*

THE STORY OF RICE

rice steamer and empty it on the ground is the greatest insult that can be dealt a Chinese family. In Japan, rice is the most sacred thing on earth and to waste it is an unforgivable sin. The Japanese have a special deity *Inari*, the rice-bearer, whose shrines dot the Japanese rural

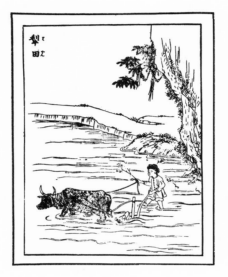

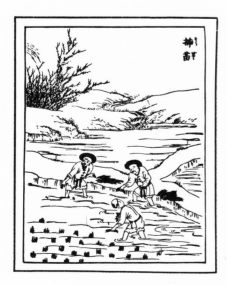 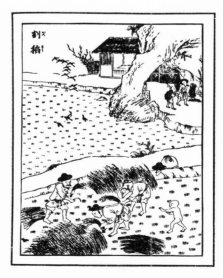

Chinese Rice Cultivation, from old Chinese engravings.

THE STORY OF RICE

landscape. There is not a village or hamlet which does not have its Inari shrine. The most popular folk-festival, the *Hatsuuma,* is held before these shrines on the 12th of February to pray for a good crop of rice. In feudal days, salaries, allowances and retainers were paid in rice

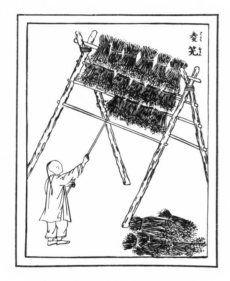 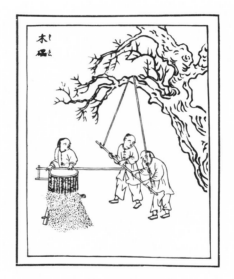

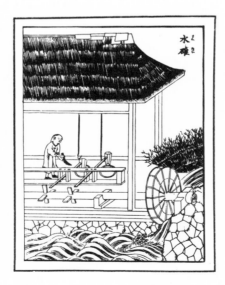 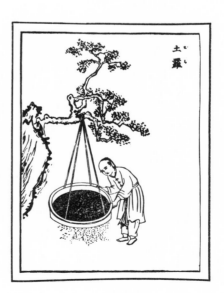

Chinese Rice Cultivation, from old Chinese engravings.

THE STORY OF RICE

instead of money. *Daimyos* or major barons received from 50,000 to 1,000,000 *koku* of rice (one *koku* was 4.9 bushels); *Shomyos* or minor barons from 10,000 to 50,000 *koku,* and retainers from a few hundred to 2,000. Imported rice was well known in the Occident long before it was cultivated in many European countries. Its name in all western tongues (*riso* in Italian, *reis* in German, *riz* in French, *arroz* in Spanish and *rice* in English) is derived from the Greek *oriza* — of Oriental origin. The first rice was introduced to North America in the year 1693, when a trading vessel from Madagascar accidently put into the harbor at Charleston, South Carolina. A small bag of Malayan *paddy* or seed rice was on board. The captain sold this little bag to a Charleston merchant and its contents became the ancestors of all the rice in the Carolinas. The Chinese and the Japanese drink an alcoholic beverage brewed from rice. The Chinese drink is called *samshu,* from *san* — three, trice, and *shao* — fire, distilled. The Japanese brew is named *sake,* from *sasake* — bamboo smell. According to an old Chinese legend, a flock of sparrows once picked some grains of rice to store for the winter in a piece of bamboo. But the autumn rains came and the tube was flooded. The rice fermented and rice wine was the result. Hence, the Chinese ideograph for *samshu* consists of the ideographs of bird and water. *Wild rice,* sold as an expensive table delicacy, is not rice, but the grain of a tall, aquatic, North American Grass *(Zizania aquatica),* which was formerly gathered by the Indians as food.

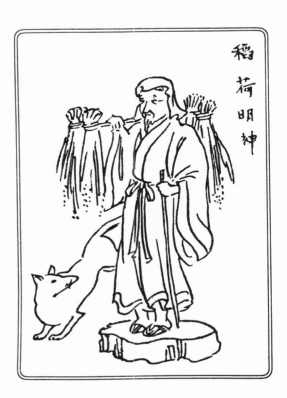

Inari, the Rice Bearer, from an old Japanese engraving.

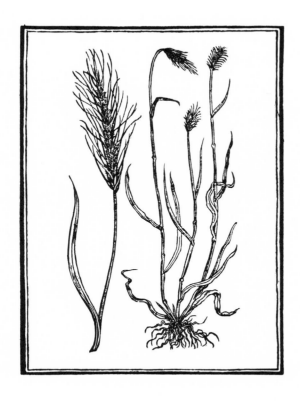

THE STORY OF RYE

The rye *(Secale cereale)*, native to western Asia and the Near East, is the hardiest of all cereal grasses and can be cultivated in soil too poor for any other grain crop. In the United States and Canada, some rye is milled into dark flour for rye bread which is well liked in large parts of North America. Because it furnishes an excellent malt, the largest part of the rye crop in Canada and the United States is used for distillation in the manufacture of liquors. In Europe the bulk of the rye crop is ground into dark flour for black bread. However, on many parts of the continent, black bread is regarded as a sign of poverty.

Rye, from Mattioli's COMMENTAIRES, *Lyons, 1579.*

THE STORY OF WHEAT

The common wheat *(Triticum vulgare)*, native to the prehistoric, untilled plains of Asia, is the oldest grain cereal known to man. It was cultivated by the Stone Age man of the Neolithic period and the Alpine lake-dweller of the Bronze Age. In ancient times wheat was the symbol of every god or goddess of harvest, from the Hittite *Ibritz* and the Egyptian *Nepri* to the Greek *Demeter* and the Roman *Ceres*. Second only to rice, wheat is today the most widely used cereal for human consumption. It is the chief food crop of the western world, from the bread-basket of the Ukraine to the grainbelts of Canada and the United States.

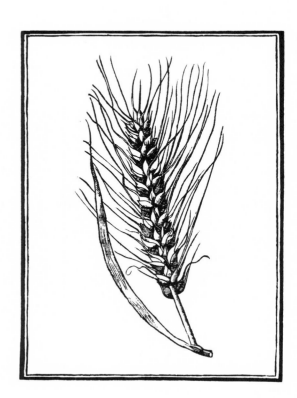

Wheat, from Mattioli's COMMENTAIRES, *Lyons, 1579.*

THE STIMULANTS

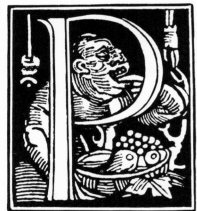

ARTS OF OUR daily food supply are not food and drink in the strict sense, but are actually stimulants. In addition to necessary food plants, man has developed other plants which give him not only nourishment but stimulation. The *caffeine* in the coffee beans and cola nuts, the *theine* in tea leaves, the *theobromine* in cocoa beans, the *nicotine* in tobacco, the alcohol in beer, wine, whiskey and untold hundreds of beverages made from every available vegetable source that lends itself to fermenting, brewing and distilling, are all stimulants. Stimulants are chemical agents or drugs which invigorate and increase some vital functional activity of the body. Their action is usually temporary and they are considered among the most valuable and important medicines; but due to their strength and sometimes poisonous properties, their effects, when misapplied, may be very serious. The term stimulant is derived from the Latin *stimulare* — to incite, to goad, to provoke. A cup of coffee, tea or cocoa, a glass of whisky or wine, a bottle of beer or a cola drink, even a bar of chocolate, are all stimulants. From the day in remote history when the first man chewed a tea or coca leaf, a betel or cola nut, a coffee bean or a fermented grape and found himself elated and vigorous, stimulants became, like food and drink, part and parcel of man's daily needs. Throughout the centuries, state and church authorities, groups of vigilantes and zealots everywhere have tried

THE RISE OF THE STIMULANTS

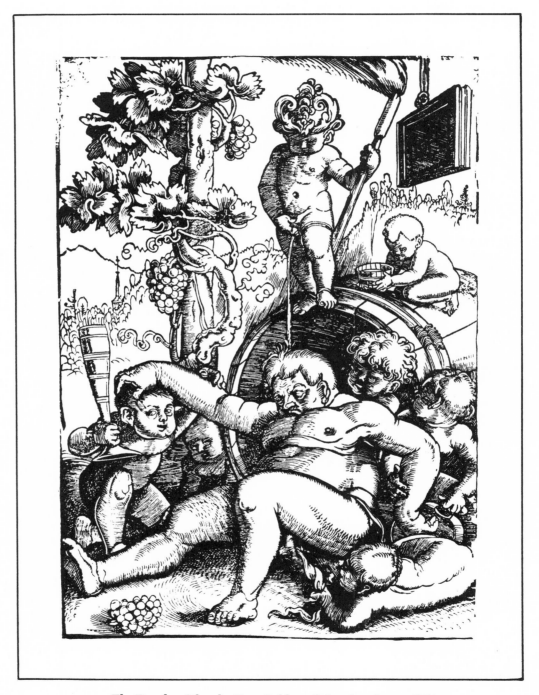

The Drunken Silen, by Hans Baldung Grien, Strasbourg, 1510.

THE RISE OF THE STIMULANTS

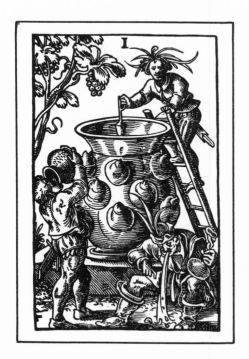
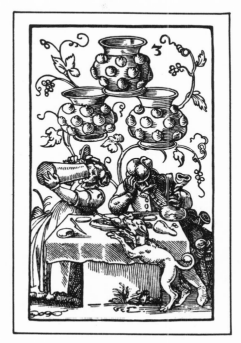
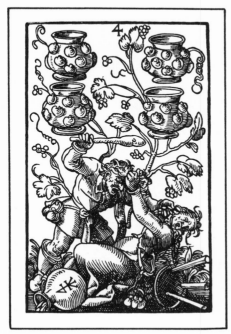
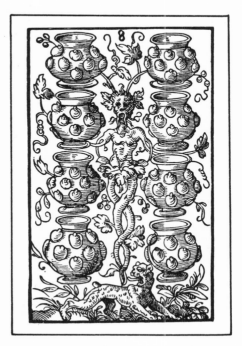

Playing Cards, from Amman's CHARTA LUSORIA, *Nuremberg, 1588.*

THE RISE OF THE STIMULANTS

to fight the use of stimulants with such weapons as scorn and ridicule, taxes and penalties, prohibition and punishment. Their efforts have been without any lasting results. In our modern hectic age, many stimulants have become necessities, and may be considered among the few luxuries available to rich and poor alike. The leading industry of many countries is to be found in the production of stimulants which frequently provide the backbone of agricultural, industrial, commercial and financial stability. It is difficult to imagine the world today without coffee and tea, without chocolate and tobacco, without coca, betel and cola, and without beer, wine, whisky or a stimulating drink of any kind. Stimulant alkaloids, as caffeine, theine, and theobromine have found widespread use as drugs in the treatment of disease, as have the numerous alcoholic beverages which doctors recommend in a variety of treatments. The alcohol used for stimulants has also found use as a base for all sorts of liquid medicinal preparations, both internal and external. New stimulants are discovered from time to time and developed in one or another part of the world. But many of these new discoveries are too dangerous to use, and only a few of them are enjoying a limited local distribution. Most consumers prefer holding on to their time-honored smokes, chews and tested traditional beverages.

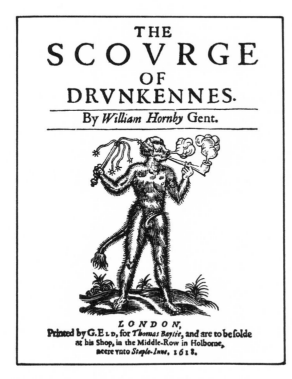

Title Page, from Hornby's SCOURGE OF DRUNKENNESS, *London, 1618.*

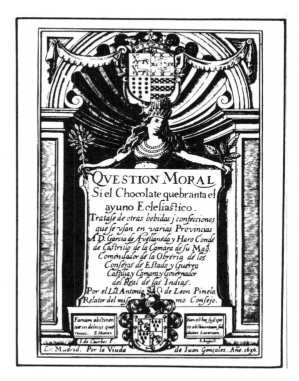

Title Page, from Leon Pinelo's QUESTION MORAL, *Madrid, 1636.*

THE RISE OF THE STIMULANTS

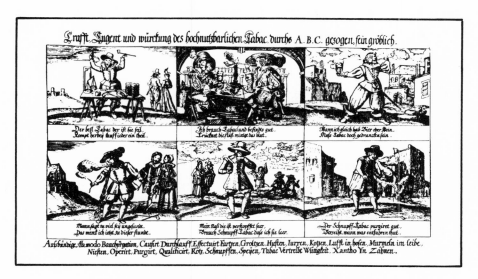

Satyric Handbill Against Tobacco, Germany, 1640.

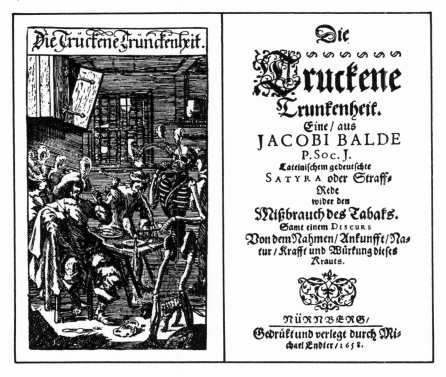

Title Page, from Balde's DIE TRUCKENE TRUNKENHEIT, *Nuremberg, 1658.*

THE STORY OF BEER

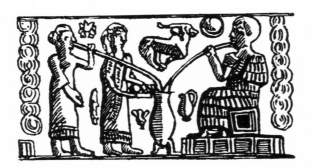

Beer-sipping Courtiers, from a Babylonian seal of Hammurabi, 1913 B.C.

It is impossible to fathom when and where the art of brewing beer was invented, for the earliest known historical records show this beverage as having already been in general use. It is believed that the knowledge of brewing beer from fermented grain is as old as that of making wine from fermented grapes. It may very well be that on a day far back at the dawn of agricultural history, in a time of famine, man opened one of his barley granaries and found his hoard in a fermented state. Short on food, he tried to boil this mushy mess and discovered to his astonishment that the resulting brew not only gave him his necessary nourishment but also induced a pleasurable exhilaration. Brewing *barley-wine* seems to be one of the oldest industrial arts of man. Brewing was already practiced about 5000 B.C. in predynastic Egypt and ancient Chaldea. An Egyptian papyrus reports that in 3400 B.C. a barley-wine tax was collected in the city of Memphis on the Nile. The oldest known recipe for barley-wine was found inscribed on a Babylonian cuneiform library brick (2800 B.C.), and the first mention of a public beerhouse on a Babylonian clay-tablet (2225 B.C.). In the time of Hammurabi, King of Babylon (1955-1913 B.C.), barley-wine was sipped by the high dignitaries of the court through golden tubes from a community vessel, as shown in the embossing on one of the king's seals. The ancient Egyptians, who knew a lot more than we realize, produced a barley-wine preserve in 1300 B.C. Barley was placed in earthenware vessels and buried in the ground until germination began; it was then finely crushed, made into a dough, formed into loaves, baked until a dark-brown malted crust developed and then sun-dried. This simplified transport by caravans through desert regions. At the point of destination, the dehydrated beer-cakes were soaked in water, until fermentation took place. The result was a sort of acid beer which is still made the same way today by the Egyptian *fellahin* for their own private use. Throughout the changing times, beer was brewed in every agricultural region of the Near East and the West. In 700 B.C. it was brewed by the Hebrews and the Armenians and, at the same time, the Greeks learned from the Egyptians the art of brewing their own barley-wine, called *zythos*. In 400 B.C. the Romans acquired from the Greeks the knowledge of brewing their *cerevisa*. Julius Caesar's legions, whose main beverages were vinegar and beer, propagated the art of malting, fermenting and brewing in all their conquered lands, from Iberia and Gaul to Germania and Brittania. In the first century of the Christian era, beer was brewed everywhere in western Europe; the Spanish

THE STORY OF BEER

brewed their *ceria,* the French their *biere,* the Teutons their *bior,* the Britons their *courmi,* and the Hiberni Irish their *coirm* (which is the ancient name of ale). Beer became more and more important as an official beverage and in 200 A.D. brewing was the prerogative of the Allemani priests, and later became the domain of the Christian monks. In 438, the *Senchus Mor,* Book of the Ancient Laws of Ireland, gave strict regulations for the growing and malting of barley, and the brewing of beer. In the 7th century, ale was the official beverage served in the Saxon councils. In 800, Charlemagne gave exact directions on how beer should be brewed for his court, and Gorm the Old, ruler of the Danes, introduced his subjects to the art of brewing in 860. Ottokar II, King of Bohemia, directed the establishment of the first official state brewery at Budweis, Bohemia in 1256; and in 1268 Louis IX, King of France, issued a law to secure the purity of beer and to protect the brewers. In 1375, Charles IV, King of Bohemia and Holy Roman Emperor, founded at Dobrow, near Pilsen, the oldest, still operating brewery in the world. The first brewery in Austria was erected in 1384 at Vienna. According to Germanic legend, Gambrinus, the personification of brewing and beer, was a mythical Flemish king who allegedly invented hop beer. In reality the name Gambrinus is a mispronunciation of the name *Jan primus* — Jan I, Duke of Brabant, who died in 1294, and was patron and protector of the Flemish Brewers' Guild. The hop plant *(Humulus lupulus)* is a climbing vine of the mulberry family, growing wild since ancient times in Europe, Asia and America. From early antiquity its young shoots were eaten as a vegetable, and its dried cones used for their slightly narcotic effect to provide a sedative against mania, toothache, earache and neuralgia. Their bitter flavor was believed to provide an effective tonic and stomachic. Hops were actually cultivated in Europe for flavoring malt liquors since the 9th century, long before Gambrinus lived. The skilled brewers of the Middle Ages were mostly the monks in their monasteries, but, in the 16th and 17th centuries, more and more commercial breweries were erected and the consumption of beer rose to such proportions that, in 1643, under Charles I, the first English excise tax was imposed on ale and beer. The first beer-brewing efforts in America were those beers brewed

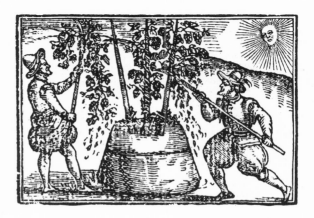

Hoppe-garden, from Scot's A PERFITE PLATFORME, *London, 1576.*

THE STORY OF BEER

privately in well-to-do households for personal consumption along with beers brewed by government licensed tavern-keepers for their own public houses. In 1637, the first brewery on a commercial basis was licensed by the Massachusetts Bay Colony to a Captain Sedgwick, but his license was revoked in 1639 on the grounds that it constituted a monopoly. A subsequent law restored to all tavern-keepers the right to brew their own beer. In 1638 the colony of Rhode Island licensed the first communal brewery under the management of Sergeant Baulson. In colonial America the position of public brewer and licensed innkeeper became an exalted one since only highly respected men of exemplary character and moral standing could obtain the right to brew and dispense beer. In 1644, Mynheer Jacobus, first burgomaster of New Amsterdam, opened the first brewery and beer-garden in that Dutch colony. William Penn brewed and sold beer at Pennsburg, Pennsylvania. Patrick Henry of Virginia was the son-in-law of an inn-keeper. In pre-revolutionary days, the British became very suspicious of brewers and inn-keepers. They considered public houses and taverns the hot-beds of revolutionary ideas, and rightly so, because the inn-keepers were, along with the printers, the driving revolutionary forces inside every patriotic organization. Taverns were the headquarters of every revolutionary fighting group. The leader of the Sons of Liberty, Samuel Adams, active head of the Boston Tea Party, was the son of a brewer and a brewer himself. The revolutionary general, Israel Putnam,

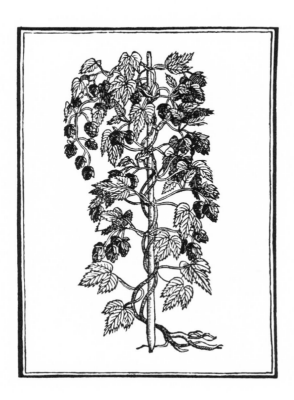

Hop Plant, from Dodonaeus' PURGANTIUM, *Antwerp, 1574.*

THE STORY OF BEER

who fought the Redcoats at Fort Ticonderoga, Bunker Hill and the Battle of Long Island, was the owner of the General Wolfe Tavern in Brooklyn, Connecticut. Captain Stephen Fay, who fought with his five sons in the Battles of Bennington and Lexington, was the landlord of the Catamount Tavern, headquarters of the Green Mountain Boys. His friend, Thomas Chittenden, first governor of the Republic of Vermont, was a brewing inn-keeper. Throughout the American Revolution, inn-keepers and taverns left their historical mark. Thus it was at Fraunce's Tavern in New York where George Washington delivered his farewell address to his officers on December 4th, 1783.

In our time the consumption of beer leads that of most other beverages in many countries. There are different kinds of beers brewed from barley: ale, named after the Anglo-Saxon *aelu* — bitter; stout, from the Middle English *stowte* — bold; porter, an abbreviation of porter's ale because it was favored by porters and laborers; lager, from the German *lager* — warehouse, because it is stored and aged for several months after brewing; bock, a corruption of *Einbeck*, the name of a German town where it was first brewed. There are beers brewed from wheat malt; the *Weissbier*, a German trade-name meaning white beer; the *Mumme*, so called because the German Christian Mumme was the first to brew this kind of beer in 1492 at Braunschweig. The Russian *kvass* is a sour beer brewed from rye flour; the Japanese *sake* and the Chinese *samshu*

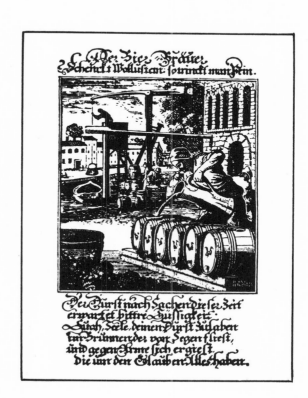

Brewer, from Weigel's GEMEIN-NÜTZLICHE HAUPT-STÄNDE, *Regensburg, 1698.*

THE STORY OF BEER

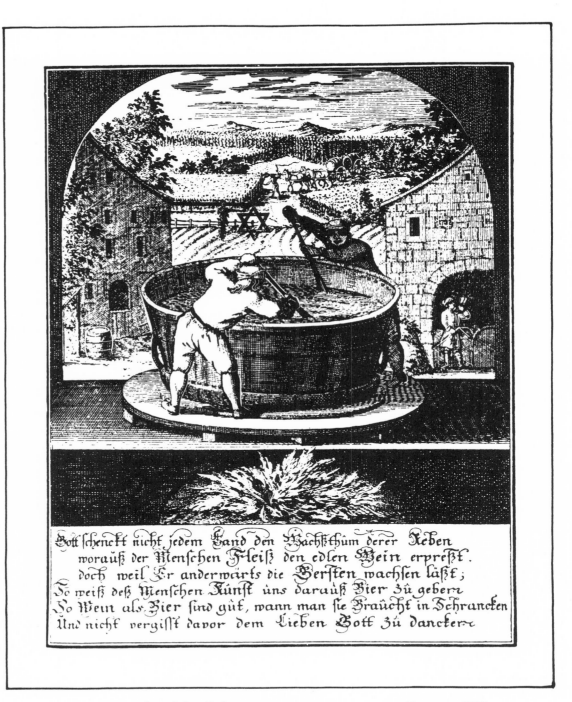

Frontispiece, from Schöpffer's TRACTAT VON BIER-BRAU-RECHT, *Germany, 1732.*

THE STORY OF BEER

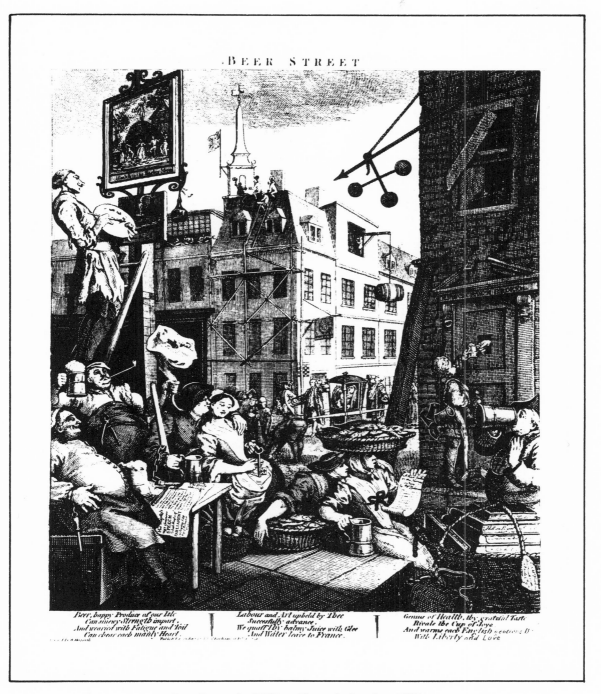

Beer Street, by William Hogarth, London, 1751.

THE STORY OF BEER

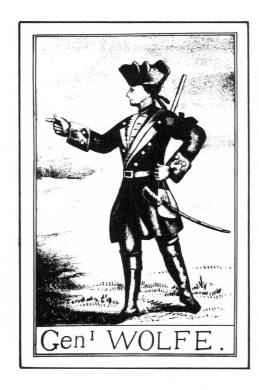

Sign, from Israel Putnam's GENERAL WOLFE TAVERN, *Brooklyn, Conn., 1768.*

Gen^I WOLFE.

are rice beers; the African *bousa* is brewed from millet, and many more beers are brewed from all kinds of grain. But there are also beers brewed from seeds, sap, twigs, leaves and the roots of all kinds of plants. The natives of Nubia and Ethiopia brew a sort of beer from the crushed seeds of the teff grass *(Eragrostis abyssinica),* and in other parts of Africa it is brewed from the fermented seeds of the spiked softgrass *(Holcus spicatus).* In the northern parts of Europe, England and America, many beer-like, undistilled beverages of very small alcoholic content are made from various kinds of plants. *Birch Beer* is made from the fermented sap of the birch *(Betula); Spruce Beer,* from a fermented infusion of bruised twigs and leaves of the spruce *(Picea),* and various spices; *Root Beer* is made from an infusion of roots, barks and herbs, such as sarsaparilla *(Smilax),* spikenard *(Aralia racemosa)* wintergreen *(Gaultheria procumbens),* and ginger *(Zingiber officinale),* fermented with sugar and yeast. In our time there are so many variations of beer and beer-like beverages that it seems impossible to name them all. In bygone days, the brewing of beer was not only a highly skilled profession but was also recognized as an art. As early as the year 1573, H. Knaust at Erfurst in Germany, published a work of no less than five volumes on that subject, with the quaint title: *On the Divine and Noble Gift, the Philosophical, the Highly Dear, and Wondrous Art to Brew Beer.* This encyclopedic work was succeeded in the centuries following by whole libraries of books and pamphlets on the subject of beer, ale and the art of brewing.

THE STORY OF THE BETEL NUT

The betel nut is the seed of the areca palm *(Areca cathecu)*, native to the warm regions of the Far East from India, Malaya and Ceylon to the Philippines and throughout the Melanesian Islands. The betel nut is the most important stimulant of the Far East, and the natives of Malaya, Madras, Penang and Singapore are so addicted to chewing betel that they would rather go without food than their steady supply of areca nuts. Betel is one of the world's leading stimulants; over one-tenth of the world's population are betel chewers. The hard kernels of the areca nut are boiled, sliced and dried in the sun. The natives take a piece of this dried nut meat, roll it with a piece of shell lime in a leaf of the betel-pepper vine *(Piper betle)* and chew this pellet like chewing tobacco. The plug has a hot and acrid taste but possesses aromatic and narcotic properties. The areca palm itself is one of the sacred plants of India and its leaves and nuts are used to adorn the images of the Vedic gods in every Brahmanic religious ceremony. It is a Hindu custom to present a betel nut to every guest as a symbol of hospitality and friendship. In Melanesia, areca nuts are used in black magic as a powerful talisman, and in marriage and religious ceremonies as a token of affection and peace. The betel nut is one of the oldest known varieties of stimulant. Betel nut chewing was enjoyed by the Chinese as early as the year 1000B.C. when it was mentioned in an elaborate herbalist manuscript on drugs attributed to the Chinese emperor, Wu-Ti.

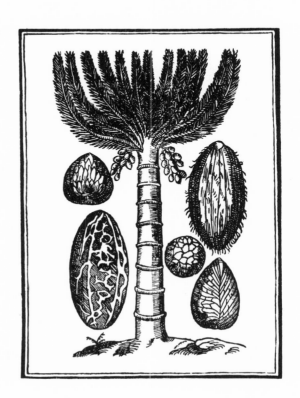

Areca Palm, from Jacobus' NEUW KREUTERBUCH, *Frankfort/M., 1613.*

THE COCA AND THE COLA

Two shrubs, the coca and the cola, from South America and Africa respectively, supplied the main ingredients for many of our soft drinks and stimulating pastilles. Their names have become household words in our daily language. Since pre-Inca times the leaves of the coca plant *(Erythroxylon coca)*, native to the mountainous regions of Peru and Bolivia, were chewed by the Indians as a stimulant and narcotic. The name is the Latinized form of the Peruvian name for the plant, *cuca*. The coca plant is the source of cocaine used since 1884 as a local surgical anesthetic. The dried nuts of the *gurru* or *kola* shrub *(Cola acuminata)*, native to the Sierra Leone and Guinea regions of western Africa, were highly valued in bygone times and used by the natives as money in local trading. Cola nuts, a source of caffeine, were chewed as a stimulant making one insensible to fatigue and hunger, and were a potent remedy for intoxication and hangover. A stimulating brew called *Coffee of Sudan*, was made from the roasted and ground cola nuts. The name is the Latinized form of the native name of the plant, *kola*. Today cola plants are grown extensively in Brazil and the West Indies to fill the growing demand of the international market for medical drugs. The narcotic coca leaves are no longer used in the manufacture of soft drinks. Other ingredients are now substituted for them and these provide equivalent stimulation without any harmful side effects.

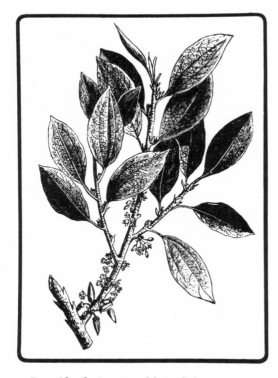

Coca Shrub, from an old English engraving.

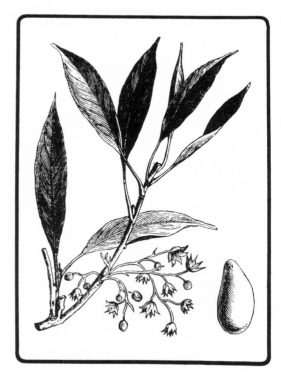

Cola Nut, from an old English engraving.

THE STORIES OF COCOA, COFFEE AND TEA

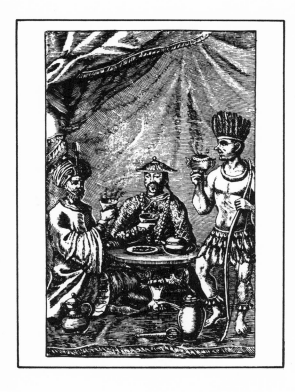

Frontispiece, from Bontekoe's DREY NEUE TRACTAT-GEN, *Bautzen, 1688.*

In the 16th century, three exotic beverages, cocoa, tea, and coffee became known in the Western World. The earliest use of these three drinks in their lands of origin is shrouded in deep mystery, but they have been used by the native peoples of these countries since ancient times. Cocoa was used by the Mayas, Aztecs, and other Indian tribes of Central and South America and the West Indies. Tea was used by the agricultural dwellers of South Asia, and coffee by the shepherds and nomads of Arabia and Ethiopia. Tea and coffee may have been known vaguely in the 14th and 15th centuries to some of the daring European land travellers to the Near and Far East. They brought samples of these plants back to Europe as unimportant oriental curiosities. Cocoa was the first of these exotic beverages to attract wide attention in western Europe; tea and coffee succeeded in short order to win the esteem of the Europeans. In 1679, Cornelius Bontekoe, professor at the University of Leyden, wrote and published the first monographs on coffee, tea and cocoa. In succeeding centuries the consumption of these stimulating drinks reached such enormous proportions in western lands that today their use has become an integral part of our daily life and it is difficult to imagine how we could get along without them. The leaves of the Paraguay Tea (*Ilex para guayensis*) yield *maté*, a brew rich in theine-caffeine. This tea enjoys little use outside of Paraguay and Brazil.

THE STORY OF COCOA

From earliest recorded history, long before the discovery of America, the natives in the West Indies and tropical countries of Latin America, bordering on the Caribbean Sea from Mexico throughout Central America and down to the coast of Brazil, made a stimulating beverage from the seeds of the *acuatl* or *chocolatl* tree. The closely packed, bean-like seeds in the cucumber-shaped pods of these trees were called *cacahuatl*, and are the source of *cacao*, whose corrupted spelling, *cocoa,* is now universally used in English-speaking countries. The botanical name of the plant is *Theobroma cacao*, from the Greek *theos* — god, and *broma* — food; hence, in free translation: *Cocoa, food of the gods.* The first reference to this new beverage was written in 1520 by Bernal Diaz, a Spanish officer who, with Hernando Cortez, visited the Aztec emperor, Montezuma II, in his palace at Temistitan, today's Mexico City. Montezuma served his guests chocolate in goblets of beaten gold. The drink was regarded as a high luxury, reserved for special occasions and eminent guests. In earlier times cocoa beans were considered so precious that they were used as money. The chocolate concoction itself was made from cocoa, the powdered beans of the chocolate tree mixed with ground annetto and anise seeds, crushed long red peppers and cinnamon. The mixture was beaten and stirred slowly over a low fire

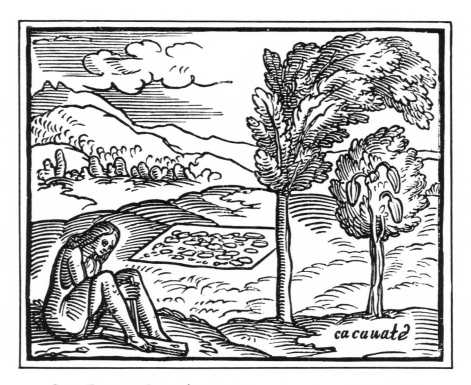

Cocoa Tree, from Benzoni's HISTORIA DEL MONDE NUOVA, *Venice, 1565.*

THE STORY OF COCOA

until it became a foamy, bubbling liquid: a sort of hot, spicy, deluxe chocolate shake. After the first beans reached Spain and Portugal, cocoa and chocolate immediately became favored food and drink items with the upper classes of society. In 1550, only thirty years after the first white men tasted cocoa in Montezuma's palace, chocolate factories of considerable size were operating in Lisbon, Marseilles, Bayonne, Turin, Genoa and many other cities throughout southern Europe. At the beginning of the 17th century, the Church tried to discourage clergy and laymen from the use of chocolate and other New World stimulants, but with no visible results. In the following centuries, chocolate trees were transplanted to Africa and the Far East to fill the steadily growing demand of Europe and North America for cocoa, chocolate and cocoa butter. Today these luxurious comestibles, once enjoyed exclusively by the ruling classes, are staple foods all over the western world, and chocolate has become an important part of the emergency rations for the armies, navies, expeditions and rescue teams of all civilized nations. The cocoa bean is regarded as one of the ideal foodstuffs in our diet because it contains carbohydrates, albuminoids and mineral matter with all three factors combined in the precise proportions required for a complete and perfect food.

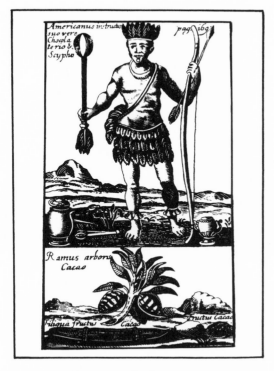

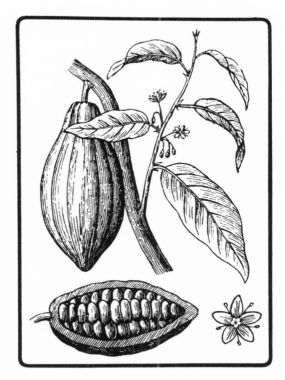

Frontispiece, from Bontekoe's DREY NEUE TRACTAT-GEN, *Bautzen, 1688.*

Cocoa Plant from Strässle's NATURGESCHICHTE, *Stuttgart, 1885.*

THE STORY OF COFFEE

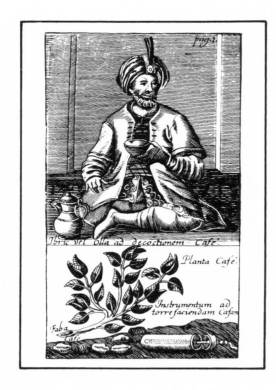

Frontispiece, from Bontekoe's DREY NEUE TRACTAT-GEN, *Bautzen, 1688.*

   The civilized world is indebted to Africa for the coffee bean *(Coffea arabica)*, native to the Abyssinian province of *Caffa*, from which its name is derived. Its early history is clouded in tradition, but it appears that the use of coffee was known to the ancient Ethiopians since time immemorial. An old Ethiopian legend claims that a goatherd by the name of Kaldi noticed that his goats, instead of drowsing in the evening, pranced around whenever they nibbled berries from a certain shrub on the hillside. He tried some of these berries himself, and became so excited over the resulting exhilaration and wakefulness, that he brought a few of the berries to the chief mullah. The chief tasted the berries and stated they were exactly what he needed to keep the faithful awake during the evening services. Coffee was not only used as a stimulant by the ancient Ethiopians, but it was also used by the Abyssinian warriors as a battle food. They mixed roasted and pulverized coffee beans with grease to form balls, and this was the only nutriment carried by raiding parties on short forays. In the 15th century, coffee beans were brought from Abyssinia across the Red Sea to Arabia which became, through its port of *Mocha* (which gave coffee its second name), the starting point that led to the universal consumption of coffee. In those days, Arabian merchants, standing at the gateway from Asia to Europe, added coffee beans from Africa to the spices and luxuries of the Orient. The Arabians, themselves, became so fond of coffee drinking that in 1470 the first public coffee houses, called

THE STORY OF COFFEE

Kaveh Khanehs, were opened in Mecca and Medina. The use of coffee spread to Damascus in Syria where in 1530 the first two coffee houses were opened under the eloquent names of the *Cafe of the Roses* and the *Cafe of the Gates of Salvation.* In 1554, coffee reached Constantinople and hundreds of coffee houses were opened up in the city on the Bosporus. At the end of the 16th century, coffee houses were a common sight in the harbor cities of the eastern Mediterranean from Venice to Cairo, and in Asia Minor from the Mediterranean Coast to Samarkand. In the middle of the 17th century, the demand for coffee rose in England and western Europe. In 1650, an Armenian from Lebanon, named Jacob, opened the first English coffee house at Oxford, under the elaborate name of the *Coffee House at the Angel at the Parish of St. Peter in the East.* In 1652, the first coffee house in London was opened by a Mr. Bowman, in St. Michael's Alley; the first French coffee house was opened in 1671 at Marseille, near the Merchants' Exchange, and the first Parisian coffee stall was put up in 1672 at the St. Germain Fair by an Armenian named Pascal. In 1683 at Vienna, after the siege by the Ottoman army under Grand Vizier Kara Mustapha was broken, the fleeing Turkish forces left hundreds of bags of coffee on the battlefield. Franz George Kolszycki, a Polish officer who distinguished himself heroically in that battle, recovered the coffee that no one else wanted, as his share of the booty. He then opened the first of the Viennese coffee houses. These European coffee houses became the

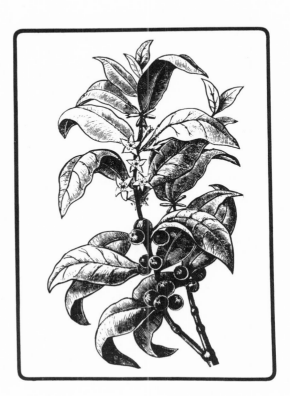

Coffee Plant, from Strässle's NATURGESCHICHTE, *Stuttgart, 1885.*

THE STORY OF COFFEE

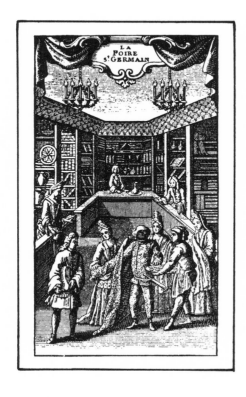

First Parisian Coffee Stall, from a French engraving, 1672.

centers of the fashionable, literary, artistic and political classes. The progress of coffee was beset with many obstacles. Religiously inclined groups denounced it as an insidiously pernicious beverage, and statesmen saw political danger in the free discussions which marked the attendance at coffee houses. The coffee houses were closed down time and again in many countries under the pressure of Church and state; heavy taxes were put on every gallon of coffee brewed, but the new beverage outlived all imposed restrictions. In North America, notwithstanding the fact that the United States is today the largest coffee consumer in the world, the institution of the coffee house never reached the social importance that it had attained, and still holds, in many countries of Europe. There were a few well-known coffee houses in the past, like John Hutchins' *The Kings Arms,* opened in 1696 on New York's Broadway between Trinity Church and Cedar Street, or the *Green Dragon* standing on Boston's Union Street for 135 years, from 1697 to 1832. But the hub of the social, political and military life of the ale, beer and whiskey drinking colonials was to be found in the inns and taverns. Until the end of the 17th century, the world depended entirely on Africa and Arabia for its supply of coffee beans. At this time all the European governments with overseas possessions tried to plant coffee in their colonies. King Louis XIV of France was the first to order the cultivation of coffee beans in the French West Indian colony of Martinique. The Dutch planted coffee in *Java* (from where the beverage

THE STORY OF COFFEE

got its third name). They also planted coffee in Sumatra and other islands of the Malay Archipelago. In 1700, the British introduced coffee into India; and the Dutch, in 1720, into Ceylon. Spanish missionaries, arriving in the Philippines from Java in 1740, brought coffee seeds along for cultivation. At about the same time, the first coffee shrubs were planted in Brazil, now the world's greatest coffee producing country. Somewhat later, coffee planting spread to Cuba, Puerto Rico, Mexico and practically all other parts of Central and South America. Today, Africa, the cradle of the coffee plant, is a comparatively unimportant factor in the great bulk of the world's coffee production. Coffee houses in their original form vanished from the American scene with the advent of prohibition. But the last two decades saw the revival of the coffee house in its old sense, on the North American continent. Thousands of refugees from European cities where the coffee house is part and parcel of the daily way of life, tens of thousands of American soldiers stationed in Europe in the occupation armies and Nato, the hundreds of thousands of American tourists, artists and students, vacationing or learning in western, central and southern Europe, acquired a taste for the leisurely life of the coffee house, and brought a desire for it to our shores. Now, progressively more coffee houses, *beatnik*, literary or just social, are springing up in cities from coast to coast all over the United States. And the best coffee today, as 150 years ago, is made after the recipe of the French diplomat, Talleyrand-Perigord: "Black as the devil; hot as hell; pure as an angel; sweet as love."

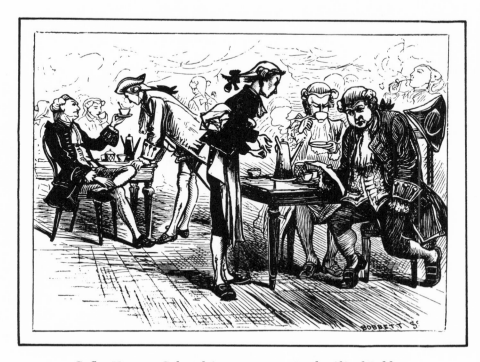

Coffee House in Colonial America, engraving by Alfred Bobbett.

THE STORY OF TEA

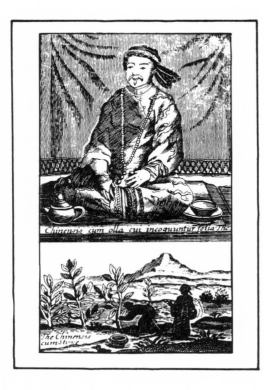

Frontispiece, from Bontekoe's DREY NEUE TRACTAT-GEN, *Bautzen, 1688.*

In China, the traditional land of flowers and legends, many a tale has been woven around the national beverage, tea. One of these ancient stories relates that an Indian prince, Bodhidharma, a pious Buddhist monk and missionary and the third son of King Kosjusva, landed in the year 510 A.D. on the coast of China to teach the doctrines of Gautama. In order to set an example of piety, Ta-Mo, the blue-eyed Brahmin, as he was called by the Chinese, vowed that he would not sleep until Bodhidharma's mission was accomplished. One day after many years of wakeful teaching, praying and meditating, Ta-Mo was overtaken by sleep. In holy wrath against the weakness of his flesh, he cut off his eyelids and threw them to the ground; but Buddha caused them to take root and to sprout a plant, the first tea shrub, symbol of eternal wakefulness, whose leaves exhibit the form of an eyelid, and possess the gift of hindering sleep. Another Chinese tradition records the discovery of the virtues of a beverage obtained by infusing tea leaves in hot water. A Buddhist hermit was replenishing a fire made from the dried branches of a tea plant, when some of the leaves fell into the vessel in which he had boiled water for his evening meal. He tasted the hot beverage that resulted — the first *"pot of tea"* — which proved to be so exhilarating in its effect that he formed the habit of using the leaves in this fashion. He imparted to others the knowledge thus accidentally gained, and in a short time the preparation of tea became the common property of all the Chinese people. According to the

THE STORY OF TEA

most reliable and authentic ancient Chinese historians and herbalists, the tea plant *(Thea sinensis)*, a member of the camelia family, is not native to China but to India. It was brought from India to China at the beginning of the 8th century A.D., during the reign of the Lyang dynasty. Tea immediately became the most popular stimulating drink for rich and poor and, in a few years time, so much tea was planted all over China that in 780 A.D. Emperor Tih-Tsung found it worthwhile to put a heavy imperial tax on the new beverage. When, in the year 805 A.D., the Buddhist missionary and saint, Dengyo Daishi, returned from the mainland to Japan to teach Buddhism to the Japanese, he brought along the seeds of the tea plant and introduced his disciples to the art of planting and brewing tea. Tea was propagated in the following centuries by Chinese traders throughout the Asiatic mainland from Mongolia to the Caspian Sea, and from the China Sea to the Persian Gulf. Tea, whose English name is derived from its Amoy name, *te,* is not merely a common stimulating beverage for the peoples of Asia, but holds a position of far greater importance among them. Like coffee in the Near East, and wine in the western world, it is the ceremonial and social drink of the Far East. The Chinese custom of serving tea to all official and private visitors, a distinct feature of Chinese social life and etiquette, originated with the Sung dynasty (960-1280), whose rulers served tea at court on all occasions. The Japanese cult of *Cha-no-Yu,* or *Ceremonial Tea,* was formulated in the

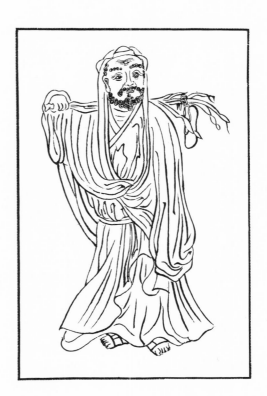

Bodhidharma, Patron of the Tea Plant, from an old Chinese drawing.

THE STORY OF TEA

BOSTON, December 1, 1773.

At a Meeting of the PEOPLE of Boston, and the neighbouring Towns, at Faneuil-Hall, in said Boston, on Monday the 29th of November 1773, Nine o'Clock, A. M. and continued by Adjournment to the next Day; for the Purpose of consulting, advising and determining upon the most proper and effectual Method to prevent the unlading, receiving or vending the detestable TEA sent out by the East-India Company, Part of which being just arrived in this Harbour:

By the Governor.

To JONATHAN WILLIAMS, Esq; acting as Moderator of an Assembly of People in the Town of Boston, and to the People so assembled:

Printed by EDES and GILL, 1773.

Report on the Boston Tea Meeting, Boston, 1773.

THE STORY OF TEA

16th century by the Samurai class as an expression of personal culture and gracious living. In 1606 the Dutch started extensive tea plantations on Java and in 1610 began to import tea into Europe. In 1640 it was already the fashionable beverage in The Hague, and in 1650, Peter Stuyvesant, Director-general of New Netherlands, introduced tea to New Amsterdam, the first importation of this beverage into North America. The English, today the largest tea consuming people in the Western World, had at that time no knowledge of tea. The first tea to reach England in 1652 consisted of only a few pounds, discovered by Admiral Robert Blake in the galleys of captured Dutch ships. The first tea was publicly sold in England in 1660 in the coffee house of Thomas Garway, Tobacconist and Seller and Retailer of Tea and Coffee, in Exchange Alley, London. The use of tea was immediately widely condemned by preachers and writers who attributed to it numerous qualities inimical to health, morals and the public order. Those outcries, however, proved futile. In the 17th and 18th centuries, the consumption of tea became so widespread and tea became so dear to the western world, that the tea trade alone with its fantastic profit margin covered all the losses of the East India Company on ships and lading lost at sea. To get out of the monopolistic grip of the East India Company, every European colonial power tried time and again to plant tea on every foot of their tropical land possessions in Africa and the Americas, without success. Tea is the only plant that can be said to have participated, even if only passively, in a revolution. The American colonists, incensed by British taxation without representation, fought the English tea imports by smuggling all the tea they needed from Holland, even though the Dutch tea cost them more than the tea from

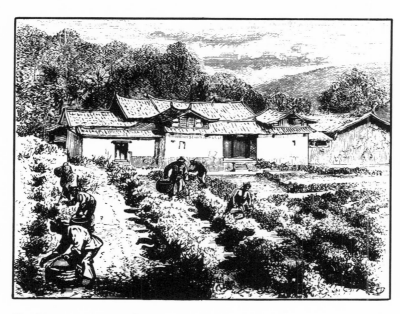

Tea Harvest, from Day's TEA, ITS MYSTERY AND HISTORY, *London, 1878.*

THE STORY OF TEA

the East India Company's ships. When the British tried to recover this lost trade by rushing ships laden with cheaper tea into Boston Harbor, a raiding party in Indian disguise under the direction of Samuel Adams, leader of the Sons of Liberty, boarded these ships on the night of December 16th, 1773 and dumped the cargo overboard. Thus, the Boston Tea Party was the first active protest against British rule in the colonies and led to the American Revolution. Anne, Duchess of Bedford, (1788-1861) is responsible for the English five-o'clock-tea. Every afternoon she suffered a "sinking feeling" which she tried to dispel with a cup of tea and cakes. In consequence, her friends soon adopted the habit of afternoon tea, elevating it into a social custom from which it developed into the familiar English institution still observed in our day. Out of a wide selection of different teas, the British developed tea-drinking into a culinary art. Among those they use are green teas from China, like *Choo-cha* — Pearl or Gunpowder tea, and *Hyson* — Blooming Spring tea; black teas like the Chinese *Congou* — Hard Labor tea, and *Souchong* — Small Sprouts tea, of which the finest is *Lapsang; Oolong* — Black Dragon tea from Taiwan; the *Pekoes* and *Orange Pekoes* — White Dawn teas like *Assam* and *Darjeeling* from India; or *Ceylon, Java, Sumatra* and *Japan* teas, and many more from other Far Eastern lands. Russia has no tea and *Russian* tea is only a trade name applied centuries ago to Chinese teas reaching Europe through Russia by camel caravans.

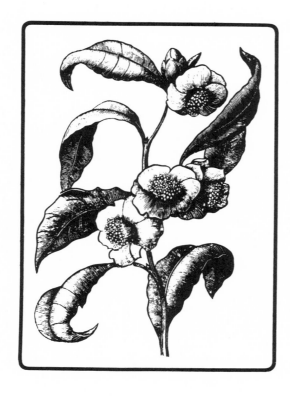

Tea Plant, from Strässle's NATURGESCHICHTE, *Stuttgart, 1885.*

THE STORY OF TOBACCO

The Mayan Rain God Smoking a Cloud-blowing Pipe, Palenque, Mexico.

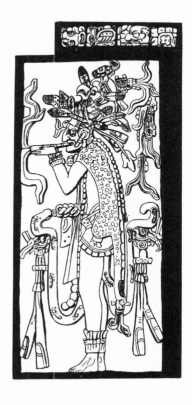

Since antiquity, chewing, sniffing and smoking dried or crushed leaves of plants, seeds and nuts has been practiced on every continent of the globe. Throughout the ages, untold hundreds of aromatic plants were burned as incense in Oriental and Occidental ceremonies and rituals; they were smoked, sniffed and chewed for medicinal purposes, used as stimulants, tonics, narcotics — or for pure sensual pleasure. But of all these various plants, none achieved either the world-wide distribution or enjoyed the favor of humanity in any way comparable to tobacco. Since early antiquity in the New World, the tobacco plant, a member of the nightshade family, has grown in two distinctive species: *Nicotiana tabacum,* native to eastern Peru and Ecuador, from which it spread throughout South America and the Caribbean; and *Nicotiana rustica,* originating in Yucatan and distributed throughout Central and North America from Panama to Florida. The smoking of the dried leaves of these plants was common practice in all of the Americas long before their discovery and exploration by the *conquistadores* and colonizers. The priests indulged in smoking in connection with religious rites, the chiefs in connection with tribal ceremonies and the medicine men employed it for purposes of both magic and fumigation. It was enjoyed by all the natives as a stimulant and narcotic. Rodrigo de Jeres and Luis de Torres, two members of the crew of Columbus, were landed on the coast of Juana (today known as Cuba) on November 2, 1492 to uncover the possible presence of human

THE STORY OF TOBACCO

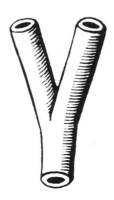

Nose Pipe, from Oviedo y Valdés' HISTORIA DE LAS INDIAS, *Salamanca, 1547.*

habitation on the island. In boarding ship again on November 5th, they mentioned in their report that the natives they encountered in the small villages carried with them lighted fire-brands of dried herb leaves rolled in a palm leaf, and that in the course of sucking on these, they puffed smoke from their mouths and nostrils with the possible intention of achieving thereby an appearance and smell that would heighten their aspect of fierceness. These two Spanish sailors were the first white men ever to set eyes on a cigar. Friar Ramon Pane, a monk who accompanied Columbus on his second voyage in 1493, related in his narrative on Hispaniola that the Indians not only smoked the leaves of this same herb, but also reduced it to a powder which they sniffed into their nostrils through a hollow cane in order to clear their heads and stomachs. This is the earliest account of snuff-taking. Nicolas Monardes reported in his *Historia medicinal*, published in 1565 at Seville, that the natives of certain parts of the New World made a dough out of ground shell lime and crushed tobacco leaves which they then formed into pea-sized pellets. After being shade-dried, these pellets were taken along on journeys through

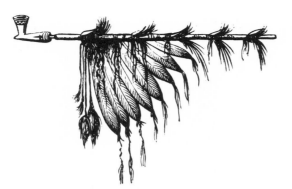

Calumet, the Peace Pipe of the North American Indians.

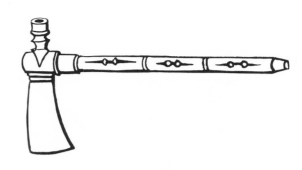

Tomahawk Pipe, the War Pipe of the North American Indians.

THE STORY OF TOBACCO

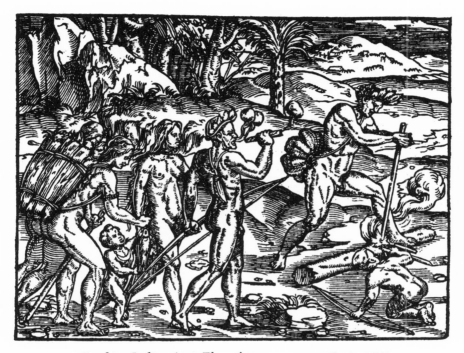

Smoking Indian, from Thevet's SINGULARITEZ, *Paris, 1558.*

arid regions; the steady sucking and chewing on these pills quenched the thirst and hunger of the travellers for many days. This is the oldest known report on chewing tobacco. The tobacco plant, which was considered to be a magical and sacred herb by the Indians, had numerous names in different parts of the Americas: *saire* in Peru, *petum* in Brazil, *zemi* in the Caribbean, *picielt* in Mexico, *uppowoc* in Virginia, and many more. But the plant was never called tobacco anywhere in the ancient Americas. Gonzales Fernandez de Oviedo y Valdes, the first chronicler of the New World, in his *Historia natural y general de las indias,* published in 1535 at Seville, named the herb erroneously after the Carib word *tabaco,* which did not mean the plant itself, but the Y-shaped tube or pipe through which the natives of the Antilles inhaled the smoke of its burning leaves. The first tobacco seeds planted in Europe for medicinal purposes were brought to Lusitania (today's Portugal) in 1558 by the Spanish physician Francesco Hernandez. In 1560 the French ambassador to the Portuguese court, Jean Nicot de Villemain, introduced the plant to France. The scientific term for the plant and its alkaloid, *nicotine,* was later derived from his name. At about the same time, Cardinal Prosper Santa Croce introduced the plant to Italy, where in his honor it was named *Erba Santa Croce.* In 1556 the first tobacco was planted in Augsburg, Germany. There was no social smoking of tobacco practiced in 16th century Europe, but smoking was already popular with captains, sailors and soldiers on ships plying between the Old and the New World. In Europe, tobacco was planted only as a strange and

THE STORY OF TOBACCO

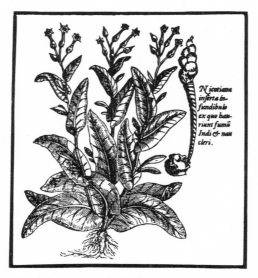

Fanciful Cigar, from l'Obel's NOVA STIRPIUM, *Antwerp, 1576.*

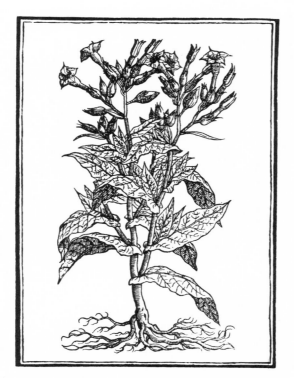

Broad Leaved Petum, from l'Ecluse's HISTORIA MEDICINAL, *Antwerp, 1579.*

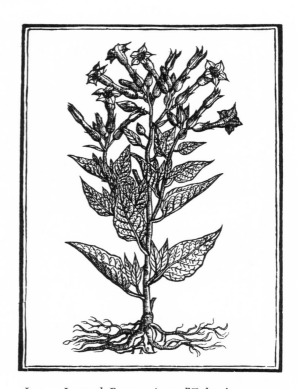

Lance Leaved Petum, from l'Ecluse's HISTORIA MEDICINAL, *Antwerp, 1579.*

THE STORY OF TOBACCO

wonderful medicinal herb, used as a cure-all for the bites of animals, snakes and insects; head-aches, colds, bruises, asthma, giddiness, rheumatism, ulcers, apoplexy and even the plague. It was called *Herba panacea* — cure-all herb, *Herba santa* — sacred herb, *San sancta Indorum* — Indian sacred cure, etc., but only its original Spanish name, *tobaco*, has remained in usage. In 1586 Ralph Lane, the first governor of Virginia and Sir Francis Drake brought the material and implements of tobacco smoking to England as a gift for Sir Walter Raleigh. It was through Raleigh's influence that the habit of *tobacco-drinking*, as smoking was called at that time, became wide-spread and fashionable. In 1600, social smoking was a common custom among men-about-town and courtiers from Spain to England, and, in that same year, the ladies of the Dutch court started sniffing perfumed tobacco. In 1604, King James I of England tried to stop the tobacco craze by publishing his famous pamphlet *Counter-blaste to Tobacco*. The amazing result of this, was that, ten years later, in 1614, the City of London alone had 7,000 shops which sold tobacco. During the Thirty Years' War (1618-1648), the soldiers of the many warring armies carried tobacco and the practice of smoking into all four corners of Europe. While most of 17th century Europe smoked tobacco in pipes, the Spanish preferred cigars. The Spanish

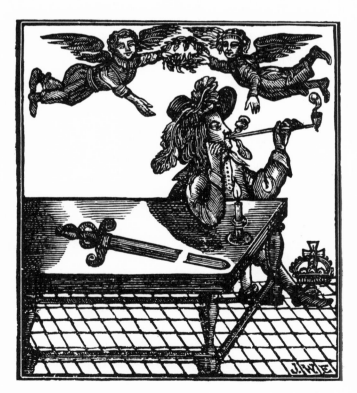

Tobacco Drinker, from Cleaveland's MELANCHOLY CAVALIER, *London, 1656.*

THE STORY OF TOBACCO

name *cigarro* was derived from *cigarra* — cicada, because the cigar resembled the body of this insect. In 1779, the first cigars were manufactured in Germany. They were made, shortly after, in France, but not before 1830 in England. In the meantime, manufacturers in Spain had been trying various types of wrappers for small *cigarillos*, using paper which had been popular as early as the 17th century. The use of these small paper-wrapped cigars, called *pepelets*, spread eastward from Spain along the Mediterranean to Turkey and the Crimean Peninsula. During the Crimean War (1854-1856), the paper-wrapped *pepelets* were introduced to French and English troops, and thanks to the returning officers, hand-rolled *cigarettes* became popular in London and Paris clubs. In 1860, British tobacco manufacturers started producing the first ready-made cigarettes. Today over sixty species of tobacco are grown all over the world, and consumed by all races, in all climates, and under all social conditions. There are some other plants whose leaves are used for smoking in considerable amount in many parts of the world. One of these, like tobacco, is of South American origin. It is the poisonous wild tree tobacco (*Nicotiana glauca*), also called by its native name *marihuana*, which was interpreted by the Spanish *conquistadores* as *Maria Juana* — Mary Jane. Later, the Spanish also applied the name *marijuana* to another ancient plant of Asiatic origin: the hemp (*Cannabis sativa*). Hemp leaves were smoked from the Asiatic mainland to the heart-lands of Africa long before the world outside of the Americas had any knowledge of tobacco. It is still smoked in India, as *bhang*, from the Sanskrit *bhanga* — hemp; in the Near East as *hashish*, from the Arabic *hashish* — hemp; and from the Sahara region to South Africa as *dakka*, the native name for hemp. In many parts of the western world, the rising trend of cigarette consumption almost appears to be reversing itself as many male smokers change back to cigars and pipes. There has, in fact, been an increase in the use of chewing plugs and snuff.

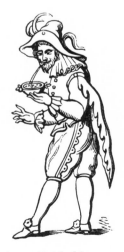

Quid Chewer, from Fairholt's TOBACCO, *London, 1859.*

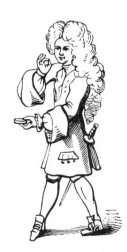

Tobacco Snuffer, from Fairholt's TOBACCO, *London, 1859.*

THE STORY OF WHISKY

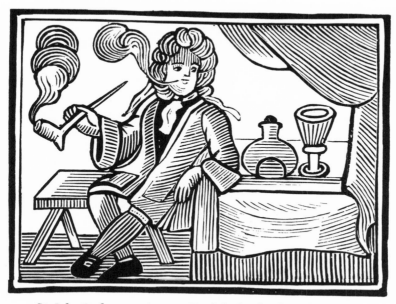

Sir John Barleycorn, from an English chapbook, 18th century.

The origin of grain liquor is shrouded in the mists of antiquity and no knowledge of its earliest existence has come down to us. The distillation of spirits from fermented grains may have started in Asia, where nearly all cereal grains originated. The ancient Egyptians believed that grain spirits were the gift of Osiris, but it is known that at least as early as 800 B.C. in India and China, grain liquor, called *arrack,* was distilled from fermented rice and *jaggery,* the coarse sugar of the sugar-palm. How the knowledge of grain distillation reached Ireland and Scotland is mysterious, but it seems possible that seafaring Arab traders roaming through the Mediterranean and along the Atlantic Coast up to Britannia in search of tin, propagated the art of distilling fermented grain cereals. Everywhere grain spirit is called the Water of Life; in Latin *aqua vitae;* in French *eau de vie;* in Swedish *akvavit.* Even in Russian *vodka* means Little Water. Our own name for it, whisky, was originally derived from the Gaelic *uisge beatha —* Water of Life, changed to *usquebaugh, usquebae, whiskeybae,* shortened to *whiskey,* and finally to our spelling, whisky. The Scots and the Irish share the honor of manufacturing the first whiskies from malted barley. The whiskies made from different grain mixtures are of recent origin.

> "Inspiring bold John Barleycorn,
> What dangers thou canst make us scorn!
> Wi' tippeny, we fear no evil;
> Wi' usquebae, we'll face the devil."
> — *Robert Burns*

THE STORY OF WINE

The use of wine as an important foodstuff and a stimulating beverage is as old as human civilization itself. The grape vine *(Vitis vinifera),* native to Asia Minor, was cultivated at the dawn of agriculture in the Near East, and wine pressed from its grapes is one of the oldest staple products for human consumption. We find an early record of the grape, its cultivation and its wine in the Old Testament: *"And Noah began to be a husbandman and he planted a vineyard: And he drank the wine and was drunken."* (Genesis IX; 20, 21). Wine was produced in abundance in ancient Babylonia, Assyria, Phoenicia, Lydia, Syria and Palestine. An old Persian legend tells how it was discovered. Prince Jemshed, being very fond of grape juice, stored a number of goatskin bags filled with fresh juice in the cellar of his desert palace. After a time he went to one of the bags for a refreshing drink, but the juice was in fermentation, tasted foul and nauseating, and gave him a severe stomach ache. To prevent others from drinking this dangerous concoction, he had all the goatskin bags labeled as poison. A short while later, his favorite wife lost his attention and, in her grief, decided to kill herself. She went to her lord's cellar and drank one beaker after another of the stored poison; but the more she drank, the gayer she became and, in her newly-won glowing beauty and intoxicated hilarity, regained her

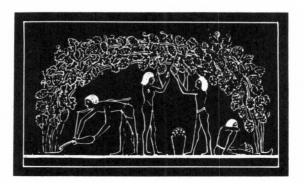

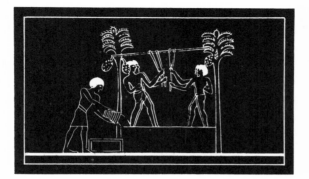
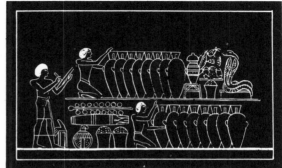

The Art of Wine Making, from an ancient Egyptian wall painting.

THE STORY OF WINE

place as favorite in the harem. She kept the secret of her revival and, every evening, took one beaker of the poison from her master's cellar. When one day Jemshed discovered that all the poison skins were empty, he investigated and found out from his favorite wife what had happened. And so he again stored grape juice for his own use and became the first wine-maker. The Egyptians of the Old Empire, technically the most advanced people in antiquity, were passionate wine drinkers. They did not produce the crude wines of the Near East, matured in goatskin bags; theirs were manufactured with great vinicultural skill. They produced four kinds of wine; white, red, black, and an especially superior northern Mareotic wine, still grown today, on the shores of Lake Mareotis, a salt lagoon near Alexandria. These ancients mastered the art of blending to improve the quality of their wines and stored them for aging in underground cellars in *amphorae,* long-necked earthenware vessels, which were carefully stoppered and sealed by the Pharoanic treasurer. From 1100 to 854 B.C., the Phoenicians, rulers of the Mediterranean, propagated grape-growing and wine-making all along the North African coast to the Iberian Peninsula (Spain and Portugal); from the islands of Cyprus, Rhodes and Crete throughout the Aegean Sea to the Peloponnesian Peninsula (Greece); and from the islands of Malta,

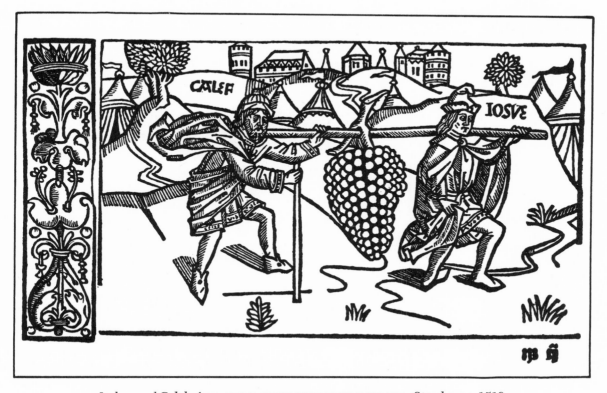

Joshua and Caleb, from BIBLIA GERMANICA DECIMAQUARTA, *Strasbourg, 1518.*

THE STORY OF WINE

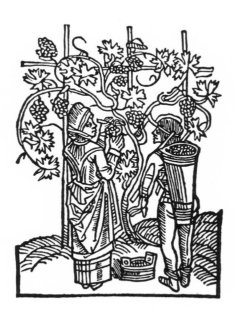

Vintagers, from Crescenzi's opus commodorum ruralium, *Speyer, 1493.*

Sicily and Sardinia to the Apennine Peninsula (Italy). In 600 B.C., the Phocians, a Greek tribe from the Corinthian Gulf, founded the town of Massilia (Marseille) on the coast of Gaul, and introduced the grape to France. Wine was so important in antiquity that all beliefs assigned its protection to special deities, as the Egyptian Osiris, the Greek Dionysus, the Roman Bacchus. In 331 B.C., when Alexander the Great, King of Macedonia, overthrew the Persian Empire at Arbela (today's Erbil in Iraq), he found the Persian vineyards in a high state of cultivation. The Chinese, contrary to popular belief, have been connoisseurs of good wine since antiquity. The grape vine was introduced into China in 126 B.C. by ambassador Chang Ch'ien on his return from a mission to the Indo-Scythians, a wine-drinking people between the Black and the Aral Seas. The Romans of the Empire, who were very fond of wine, invented for their lavish banquets the wine-cooler filled with snow which was brought down from the Apennine mountain-tops by relays of slave-runners. They also originated the custom of toasting an honored banquet guest with wine, a practice still prevailing in our time. There is, however, this small difference: the Romans, more robust than we are today, drank one glass of wine for every letter in the toastee's full name, quite a feat — in the case of TITUS FLAVIUS SABINUS VESPASIANUS. The Roman legions, in their conquest of western and central Europe, introduced wine wherever they went: in 55 B.C. under Julius Caesar to Britannia (England); under Marcus Aurelius Antonius (161-180 A.D.) to Vindobona (Vienna), from which wine was introduced to Germania (Germany); and under Marcus Aurelius Probus (276-282 A.D.) to Transleithania (Hungary). When Attila, the "Scourge of God", King of the Huns, invaded Hungary in the middle of the

THE STORY OF WINE

5th century, he became so fond of Hungarian wine that he gave the vintners around Tokay every protection. This patronage enabled the Tokay vineyards, at a time when everything in eastern and central Europe was nearly destroyed by the savagery of the Huns, to develop one of the finest strains of wine in the world. Wild vines have grown on the North American continent since time immemorial. They grew in abundance on the eastern coast when Leif the Lucky landed somewhere between Maine and New Jersey in 1000 A.D. He named the newly found continent *Vine Land*. After the rediscovery by the British, they found that these wild vines and hard grapes of North America were not suitable for producing drinkable wine. But they were so hardy that they could be used with excellent results for grafting with the more delicate vines of Europe. The London Company sent forces of French vintners and large quantities of cuttings from European vines to the colonies for grafting, and after a time of bickering by the colonial officials and petty resistance by the farmers to raising wine on their land grants, the production of wine started on North American soil. In the year 1622, the first small quantity of Virginia wine, badly matured and further spoiled by musty casks and the long sea voyage, reached England in an undrinkable state. Through special laws and bounties awarded for wine raised in colonial vineyards, production improved slowly, and wine is today a staple crop from New York to California, and from the Carolinas to Ohio. France has the distinction of having changed the age-old recipe for making wine, introducing to the world a new kind of stimulating beverage, *champagne*. The discovery was made by Dom Perigon, a Benedictine monk who died in 1715. Father Perigon, a blind man who worked in the monastery's vineyards, developed such

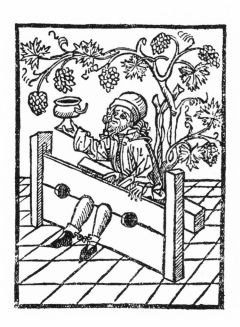

Drunkard, from Berger's SPIEGEL MENSCHLICHER BEHÄLTNIS, *Augsburg, 1489.*

THE STORY OF WINE

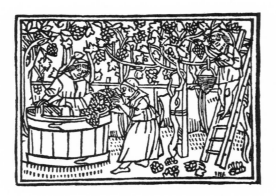

Vintagers, from Crescenzi's LIBRO DELLA AGRICUL-
TURA, *Venice, 1511*

a high taste and knowledge of the wines of different grapes and their blending, that he was put in charge of the wine cellars. He discovered there that the effervescence of fermenting and aging wine evaporated through the wool-stoppers which were dipped in oil and wax and used for wine bottles in those days. He ordered some stoppers fashioned from cork and, with a piece of

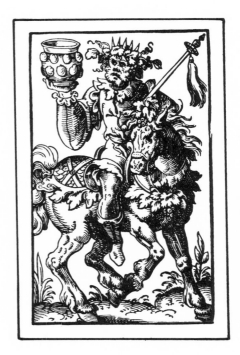

Bacchus Playing Card, from Amman's CHARTA
LUSORIA, *Nuremberg, 1588.*

THE STORY OF WINE

Coopers, from Crescenzi's LIBRO DELLA AGRICUL-
TURA, *Venice, 1511*

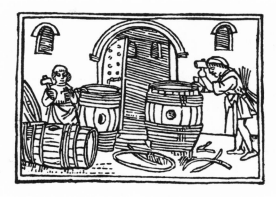

wire, secured them to the necks of the bottles. This simple change of stoppers led to the discovery of sparkling wine. Today over 1,500 different species of grape-vines are used all over the world to manufacture one of the oldest stimulating beverages of mankind, along with its aristocratic offspring, champagne. The science of viticulture, from the Latin *vitis* — the vine, and

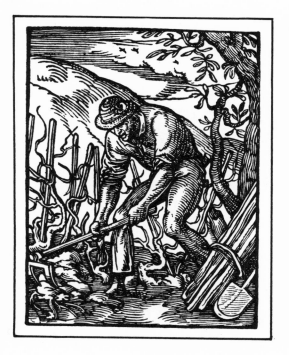

Vintager, from Amman's BESCHREIBUNG ALLER
STÄNDE, *Frankfort/M., 1568.*

THE STORY OF WINE

cultura — cultivation, also called ampelography, from the Greek *ampelos* — the vine, and *graphia* — the writing of, is today a very important subject in the curriculum of every agricultural college on the globe. There is no other plant as useful to man as the grape vine. Its fruit is used not only as the basic material for the production of alcoholic beverages, but also as an important food in itself. Grapes in large quantities are consumed fresh, dried as staple food in the form of raisins, malagas, muscatels, valentias, sultanas and currants. The grape seeds in the pulp of the wine presses offer a further yield of grape-seed oil, and the skins are used as cattle fodder. Tendrils are brewed into a medicinal tea, and the resin and sap is used as a home remedy for disorders of the kidneys and bladder. Prunings are pressed for an excellent vinegar, and leaves are pickled as a sweet-sour relish. The branches, cut off in the Fall, are burned to furnish potash and fertilizer. Today, wine is manufactured and used in nearly every land on the globe where the climate is warm enough. The Mohammedan countries are the exceptions because the Koran forbids the use of the fermented juice of the grape to all faithful Moslems.

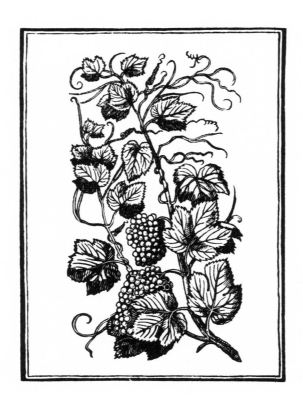

Grape Vine, from Mattioli's COMMENTAIRES, *Lyons,*
1579.

THE ODYSSEYS OF PLANTS

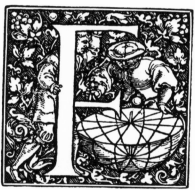

LOWERS, PLANTS AND TREES are stationary living bodies which could be choked by their own descendants growing too densely from seeds dropped in their immediate vicinity. But nature has developed all kinds of fantastic transportation facilities to enable the parent plant to distribute its seeds over wide areas for the propagation of the species. There are plants whose seeds sail through the air like the dandelion or the maple; others roll along the ground like the tumbleweed or the Rose of Jericho; some ski over the snow like the jimson weed or the locust tree; still others like the martynia or the cockle-bur ride in the fur of passing animals; some travel in the stomachs of birds like the pits of the fruit trees; and some even navigate the oceans like the coconut or the East Indian mulberry tree. But in the past the self-propagation of plants, with a few exceptions, was severely limited by snow-covered mountain ranges, by the arid sands of vast deserts, or by large bodies of water. It took the ingenuity and tenacity of man to span these mountains, deserts and oceans, and to transplant the seeds of many plants in new soils of far-away regions and continents with results that were sometimes amazing.It was not long before plants once unknown on these continents became so abundant that their crops not only supplied enough staple food for the whole population but also an important new export item for these regions.

THE STORY OF THE BANANA

The native home of the common banana *(Musa paradisiaca),* a palmlike plant with large clusters of edible fruit, was in all probability the humid tropical region of southern Asia. The over-population and the exhaustion of the soil in these parts of south Asia at the time of Christ were the cause of great migrations of south Asian people to the Indonesian and Pacific Isles. They carried the banana with other agricultural products to their new island homes: Sumatra, Borneo, Java, Formosa, the Philippines, Hawaii and the Easter Islands. Arab traders introduced the banana from Indonesia to Madagascar, East Africa and the Near East. In 650 A.D., the plant came to northern Egypt with the Mohammedan conquerors, and from there along the Mediterranean coast to West Africa. In 1460, Portuguese navigators and slave traders carried the banana to the Canary Islands along with the Negro slaves from Guinea. According to Oviedo y Valdes in his first natural history of the New World, the banana was introduced to the Americas in 1516 by Friar Tomas de Berlanga, who brought the first plant from the Canary Islands to Santo Domingo. In 1531, the Spanish *conquistadores* took the banana to Mexico, and during the 17th and 18th centuries it was cultivated in practically all of tropical America.

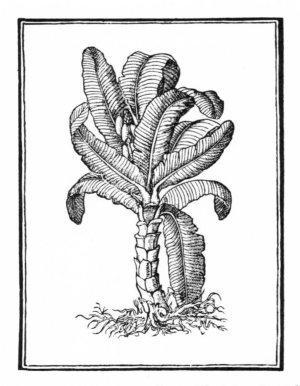 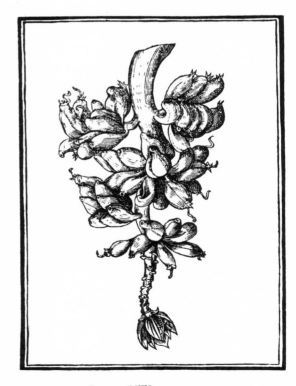

Banana Plant, from Mattioli's COMMENTAIRES, *Lyons, 1579.*

THE STORY OF THE BREADFRUIT TREE

Throughout the islands of Polynesia there is no tree so valuable as the breadfruit tree *(Artocarpus altilis)*. The huge fruit of this tree (the size of a man's head) with its sweet, starchy, seedless pulp is the staple food of the native population in the Pacific Islands for the eight months it is in season. Roasted in its thick skin between hot stones, the pulp of the breadfruit achieves the consistency and taste of freshly baked bread. The earliest account of the bread-fruit came from Captain William Dampier, English navigator, explorer and pirate, on his return in 1688 from Guam, one of the Ladrone Islands. Captain James Cook, English navigator who explored the Pacific in 1770-80, reported in such glowing terms about the value of the breadfruit that the British government decided to transplant young breadfruit trees to her American colonies. When *H.M.S. Bounty* sailed in 1786 from Tahiti, Captain William Bligh's sole commission was to bring breadfruit trees from the Society Islands to Jamaica in the West Indies. The fate of the Bounty on this trip is well known, but a later expedition was more successful, and today the breadfruit is a valuable crop from southern Florida to Brazil providing the natives around the Gulf of Mexico and the Caribbean Sea with an all important staple food.

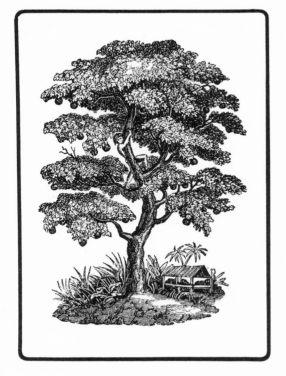 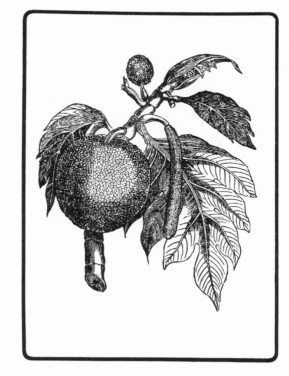

Bread Fruit Tree, from an old English engraving, 1832.

THE STORY OF THE COCONUT

One of the most versatile world travellers is the fruit of the coconut palm *(Cocos nucifera)*, native to the numerous islands dotting the southern Pacific. This fruit has needed no help from human beings in crossing and recrossing the oceans, and it grows today on the sandy coast of every continent and island in tropical waters. Well adapted by nature for sea travel, the coconut has a thick, fibrous husk which makes it buoyant in water; a hard, leathery, watertight shell, and a hollow center, partly filled with a milky fluid. Its name is derived from the Portuguese *coco* — grimace, because it resembles a grinning human face. The coconut palm, growing along sandy coastal strips, drops its ripe nuts which are swept by the tides into the ocean, thus starting their long journey to whatever faraway shores the currents may lead them. Tossed by the waves upon a suitable beach, a plant emerges through the soft eye of the nut, taking root and growing into a new coconut tree. The coconut palm is the staff of life and general provider for the island peoples of the tropics. According to the South Sea proverb: *"He who plants a coconut tree plants food and drink, vessels and clothing, a habitation for himself and a heritage for his children."* The coconut is an important commercial crop on all the tropical islands. The sun-dried meat of the cracked nut, called *Copra*, from the Hindu *khopra* — skull nut-shell, is exported to all western lands as raw material in the production of oil, margarine and soap.

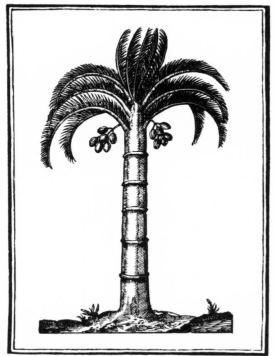

Coconut Palm, from Jacobus' NEUW KREUTERBUCH, *Frankfort/M., 1613.*

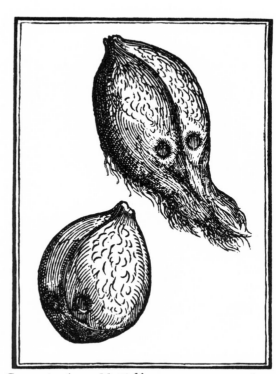

Coconuts, from Mattioli's COMMENTAIRES, *Lyons, 1579.*

THE STORY OF COTTON

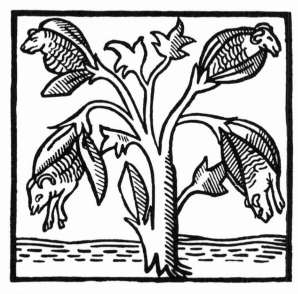

The Lamb Tree, from Maundevile's VOIAGE AND TRAVAILE, *London, 1725.*

The cotton *(Gossypium)*, a member of the mallow family, is one of the few plants which, by some quirk of nature, has grown since ancient times on two unconnected, antipodal continents of the globe, south Asia and Central America. Neither region can claim priority for the raising of cotton, or the weaving of cotton cloth. In the Hindu mythology of creation, *Manu* refers to the extensive cultivation of the cotton plant and the spinning and weaving of cotton fabrics in ancient India long before the year 800 B.C. On his triumphal return from India in 323 B.C., Alexander the Great brought cotton to Asia Minor. In 300 B.C. the agricultural planting of cotton was already practiced in Upper Egypt and, at the same time, cotton was grown as a decorative garden plant in ancient Greece. In 600 A.D. cotton reached China and Korea in its travels from India to the Far East. In the year 789 A.D., a Chinese junk laden with cotton seed was driven from its course by ill winds and shipwrecked on the Japanese coast. Its seed load started the propagation of cotton throughout Japan. The Saracens, who conquered Sicily in 821 A.D., introduced the cotton plant to this island. In the year 912 A.D., the Caliph of Cordova, Ab-der-haman III, established the first cotton plantation in Spain and in 1350 the Turks brought cotton to the Balkan Peninsula. In the Dark Ages, when all of Europe was in the grip of complete ignorance, every weird tale told by adventurers returning from unknown lands was believed as gospel. Land-travellers coming back from Samarkand reported that there existed in Tatary and the lands beyond Cathay (China), a vegetable lamb tree, called by the natives *barometz*. The fruit of this tree was said to resemble a lamb, with feet, hooves, ears and woolly head. The hanging heads of these lamb-fruits were believed to feed on the surrounding

THE STORY OF COTTON

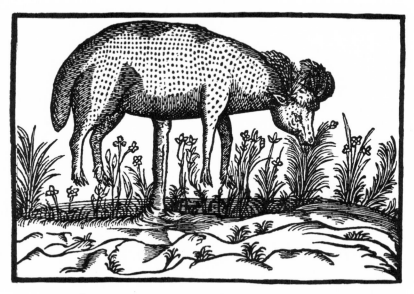

The Barometz, from Duret's HISTOIRE DE PLANTES,
Paris, 1605.

grass and, when the grass was eaten or cut away, the plant perished. The woolly tufts of these lamb-heads were gathered by the natives who spun them into fine threads which were woven into beautiful Indian fabrics and brought to the west for centuries by Arab traders as one of the most precious items of goods from the Orient. The Arabs called this fabric *al-quton,* which changed to the Spanish *algodon,* the French *coton,* the German *kattun,* and finally to the English *cotton,* both for the plant and the fabric. Notwithstanding the fact that cotton was raised and spun all along the Mediterranean Sea, the belief in the Far Eastern lamb tree haunted the herbals of outstanding naturalists for centuries to come. On the other side of the globe, long before the white man came to the Americas, cotton was cultivated by the ancestors of the Aztecs, Mayas, Columbians and Incas. The spinning of cotton thread and the weaving of cloth was a highly developed native art. Cotton was woven by the Indians from dyed threads into fabrics of every degree of fineness from muslin to velvet. Some of these fabrics were interwoven with animals' hair and birds' feathers, giving the material unusual appearance and delicate beauty. When Christopher Columbus landed in 1492 on the island of Hispaniola, he found the natives wearing colorful cotton robes. This was one of the reasons for his belief that he had reached India, the land of cotton fabrics. Bernal Diaz, accompanying the first unsuccessful expedition into Mexico under Hernandez de Cordova, reported after the Spanish withdrawal from Yucatan in 1517, that the Aztec warriors whom they encountered, were protected with an efficient armor of long, heavy coats made from a thickly woven cotton. In 1520, the Portuguese navigator, Ferdinand Magellan, found that the Brazilian Indians wore cotton fabrics. In 1619,

THE STORY OF COTTON

cotton was planted by colonists along the rivers in Virginia, and the first Negro slaves were imported into North America to till the new plantations. Throughout the 18th century, the Spanish West Indies and Portuguese Brazil were the leading cotton producing and exporting centers of the New World. Cotton was at that time not too important in the agriculture of the North American colonies. Only in 1793, when the American inventor, Eli Whitney, created his saw-toothed cotton gin, did cotton planting in North America get its biggest boost. This was a simple machine for the extraction of the seeds from raw cotton. Today cotton is the most important crop in the *cotton belt,* the region in the southern part of the United States, extending from Florida to Texas, making the United States the largest cotton producer in the world, not only for cotton fiber, but also for the manufacture of cotton-seed oil. Though synthetic fibers have made inroads into the various uses for cotton today, the industry is still more than able to hold its own through the development of various industrial uses, new foreign markets, and through the new chemically treated cotton fibers, which have given cotton the same useful characteristics as the most highly developed of the synthetic fibers.

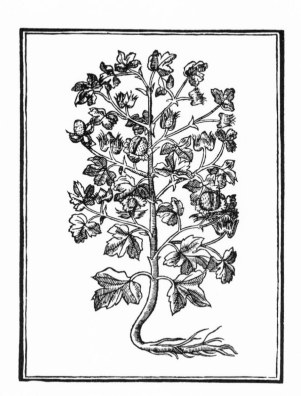

Cotton Plant, from Mattioli's COMMENTAIRES, *Lyons, 1579.*

THE STORY OF PAPER

Hieroglyphic Symbol for Papyrus, emblem of ancient lower Egypt.

The oldest form of writing paper made from plants was the *papyrus* of ancient Egypt. Its source was the famous paper reed *(Cyperus papyrus)*, a waterplant which grew in abundance in the delta and on the marshy banks of the lower Nile. The papyrus plant was, in ancient Egyptian belief, the symbol of protection from crocodiles and it became the hieroglyphic emblem of lower Egypt. The same protective symbolism is noted in Biblical legend which says

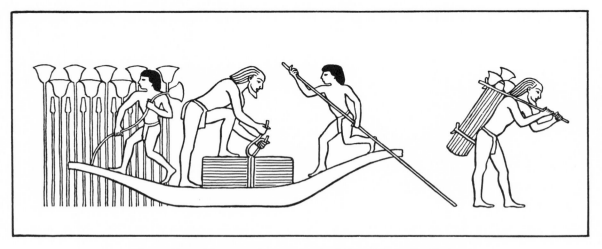

Harvesting of Papyrus, from an ancient Egyptian wall painting.

THE STORY OF PAPER

Bamboo, the Earliest Source of Paper, from an old Chinese drawing.

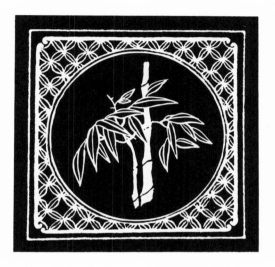

that the papyrus provided the material from which the basket for the infant Moses was constructed. The process of making paper from papyrus was invented in 2200 B.C., and its practice lasted till the 4th century A.D. This papyrus paper was manufactured by removing the outer rind from the reed of the plant. The pith was then sliced into thin strips and these strips were laid side by side with one or two layers put across and laminated together with the viscous

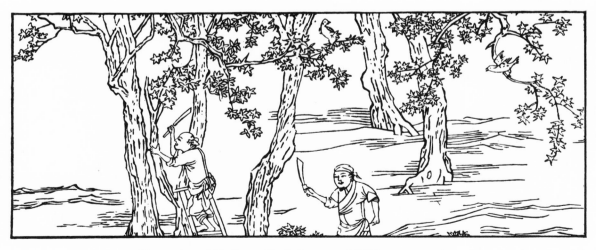

Harvesting of Mulberry Bark, from an old Chinese engraving.

THE STORY OF PAPER

sap of the plant roots as an adhesive. The resulting sheets were then pressed and dried, providing a papery product with a very fair surface for writing upon. The writing itself was done with pointed pens cut from the thinner reeds and an ink made from carbonized rush. The planting and harvesting of papyrus, the manufacture of paper, pens and ink were government monopolies in ancient Egypt. The technique of lamination, lost in the Dark Ages, was rediscovered in our time and is used today in the production of plywood. For centuries, Egyptian papyrus was an important industrial export to Assyria and other countries in Asia Minor, and to Greece and Rome, because all these countries had only bricks, copper sheets, rolls of leather, clay and wax tablets as writing materials. The papyrus was the predecessor of parchment, a writing material made from shaved sheepskin or goatskin, invented in the city of Pergamum in Asia Minor (today's Bergama in western Turkey), from which its Latin name *pergameum* — paper, is derived. Parchment displaced papyrus in Europe until the appearance of handmade fiber paper in the 12th century, a process known at that time in the Far East for more than a thousand years. In the year 105 A.D., Ts'ai Lun, the chief eunuch of the Chinese Emperor Ho-Ti, invented the art of paper-making from plant fibers. Until that time Chinese

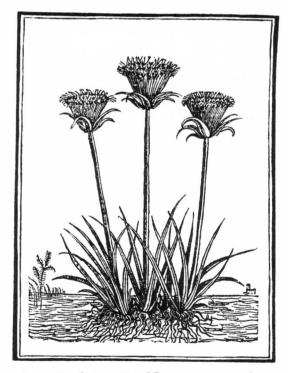

Paper Reed, from Gerald's HERBALL, *London,*
1633.

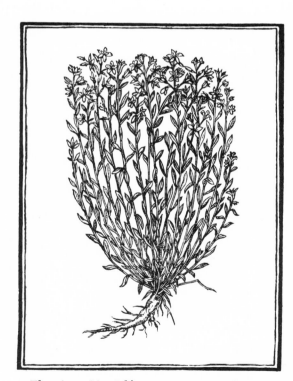

Flax, from Mattioli's COMMENTAIRES, *Lyons,*
1579.

THE STORY OF PAPER

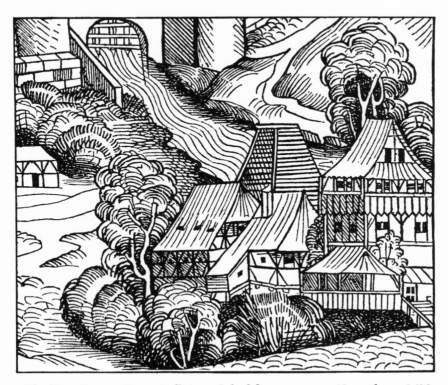

The First German Paper Mill, from Schedel's CHRONICLE, *Nuremberg, 1493.*

records were engraved on wooden tablets or painted on silk. The first raw material used by Ts'ai Lun was the fiber of the bamboo reed and the bark fiber of the mulberry tree, both plants growing in abundance in ancient China. The fiber was soaked in water, stamped in mortars to loosen it up, and to make it flexible and soft, mixed with lime and water and boiled. The resulting pulp was then poured into box-like moulds of woven cloth framed with bamboo; the water was drained off and the sheet of paper pressed and dried. In 600 A.D., the knowledge of manufacturing fiber paper had reached Korea and Japan, where not only bamboo and mulberry bark were used, but also rice straw. About 750 A.D., paper from flax fiber was manufactured in Samarkand, Uzbekistan. When the Arabian armies, returning with prisoners from their conquests in Central Asia, discovered that some of these captives knew how to make paper from plant fibers, the first paper-mill was established in 794 by Caliph Harun-al-Rashid at Bagdad, with flax fiber and linen rags used as raw materials. The Arabic Moslems built paper-mills wherever they conquered: in the year 900 A.D. in Cairo, Egypt; in 1100 in Fez, Morocco and on the isle of Sicily; and finally in 1144 at Xativa, Spain. Veterans of the Crusades carried the secret of paper-making from the Holy Land back to Europe, and the first paper-mill in France was established in 1189 at Herault, followed in 1276 by the first Italian mill at Fabriano; the first German mill was founded in 1390 by Ulman Stromer at Nuremberg. The development

THE STORY OF PAPER

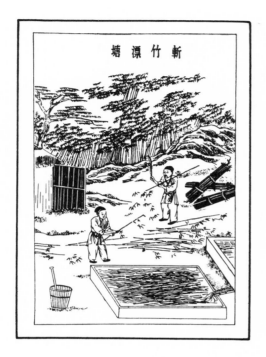
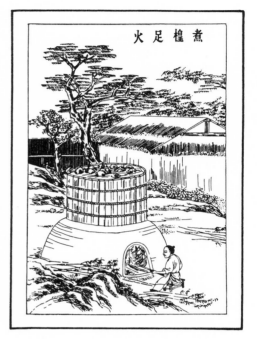
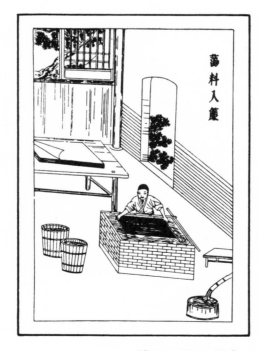
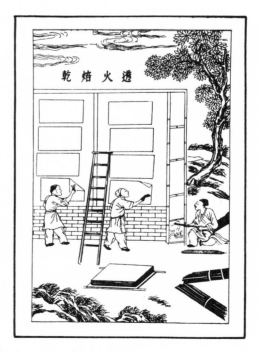

Chinese Paper Making, by Sung Ying-hsing, 1643.

THE STORY OF PAPER

of paper-making was strongly opposed by the Guilds of Parchment Makers, whose product was made by an expensive and elaborate process. They denounced rag paper as a cheap and inferior substitute for parchment and employed all possible means to prevent its use, but with constantly diminishing effectiveness. Paper-mills were built all over Europe, and John Tate, the son of London's Lord Mayor, established the first English paper-mill at Hartford in 1494. The first paper-mill in Mexico was founded in 1575 at Culhuacan by Hernan Sanchez de Munon and Juan Cornejo. In 1690 the Mennonite bishop, William Rittenhouse, and the printer, William Bradford, opened the first paper-mill near colonial Germantown, Pennsylvania. Up to that time, and for a time still to come, all the western paper-mills followed the Arabian recipe, using linen rags for the manufacture of paper. The reason was that rags from old long-used garments provided a completely soft and crushed fiber. Since printing and writing grew to enormous proportions in the 18th century, mills became famished for old rags and experimented with every kind of fiber they could find: thistles, nettles, moss, asparagus, peat, artichokes, rush, sea-weed, and hundreds more. The results were completely unsatisfactory. In 1719, the renowned French naturalist and physicist, René Antoine Ferchault de Réaumur, discovered the secret of how the Canadian paper wasp built its waterproof nest with a substance resembling paper. The wasp macerated wood slivers, sized the substance with its saliva, and spread this pulp thinly over its nest where it dried into a thin, strong paperlike sheet. The German, Jacob

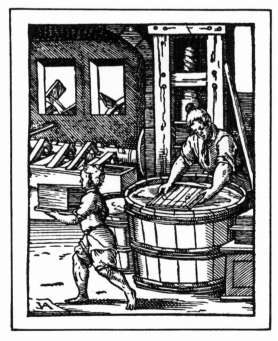

German Paper-maker, by Jost Amman,
Frankfort/M., 1568.

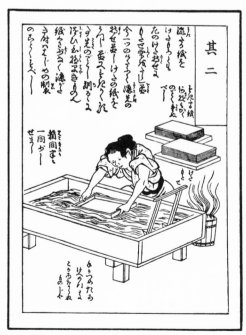

Japanese Paper-maker, by Kunihigashi Jibei,
1798.

THE STORY OF PAPER

Christian Schaffer, at the end of the 18th century, made the first experimental paper from wasps' nests. In 1799 the Frenchman, Nicolaus Louis Robert, at Essones, patented the first machine to make paper in continuous sheets. John Gilpin at Wilmington, Delaware, built the first American paper machine in 1817, producing the first machine-made writing paper in North America, consisting of a sheet 1,000 feet long and 27 inches wide. In 1827 the American potash manufacturer, William Magaw, produced, by accident, the first American paper from straw. When he lined his potash hopper with long straw it turned into a papery mass. He submitted his discovery to George Shyrock, who operated a paper mill at Hollywell Mill, near Chambersburg, Pennsylvania. Shyrock started to make straw paper on a cylindrical machine, but the wet layers of paper fused themselves into a solid board. This second accident led to the discovery of strawboard, revolutionizing the manufacture of paperboxes for all kinds of commercial goods. In 1867, the Germans, Friedrich Keller and Heinrich Volter, displayed at the exhibitions in Paris and London, a new machine for grinding wood into pulp which could be used for the manufacture of a cheap, thin paper, which is today's newsprint. The Keller-Volter display gave rise to the tremendous boom in low-priced newspaper editions that has continued to the present day.

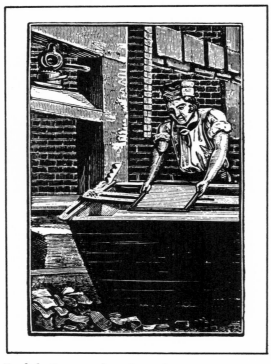

English Paper-maker, from the BOOK OF ENGLISH TRADES, *London, 1818.*

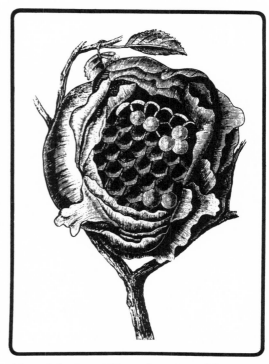

Nest of the Paper Wasp, from Strässle's NATURGESCHICHTE, *Stuttgart, 1885.*

THE STORY OF THE PEANUT

The groundnut or peanut *(Arachis hypogaea),* native to Peru and Brazil, is a vine of the pea family. Its flowers bend after fertilization and push underground where the seeds ripen in brittle, papery shells. Peanuts were cultivated extensively by the Incas and Mayas in antiquity. Spanish explorers took *arachis* seeds to Spain and Africa, from where the peanut travelled to Java, China and Japan, becoming an important food throughout Africa and Asia. African *arachis* was carried back to America on slave ships as food for the Negro slaves, which brought the peanut into complete disrepute as a food for both slaves and masters alike. Thus, in the following centuries, peanuts were cultivated in the gardens of Virginia and the Carolinas only as floral curiosities. The commercial history of the peanut in North America begins with the Civil War when Union soldiers discovered that the nuts roasted in their camp fires made excellent eating. In the years succeeding hostilities, the acreage assigned to peanut cultivation increased steadily in Virginia, the Carolinas, Georgia, Alabama, Florida, Tennessee, Texas, Arkansas and Mississippi. The American Negro botanist, chemist and educator, George Washington Carver (1864-1934), became the pioneer of peanut agriculture, and today the peanut is one of the principle food crops in the southern United States, consumed in the form of roasted peanuts, peanut butter, peanut brittle, *arachis* oil and peanut meal.

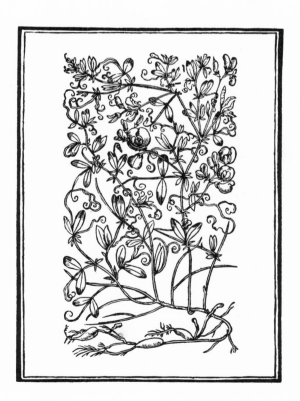

Peanut Plant, from Mattioli's COMMENTAIRES, *Lyons 1579.*

THE STORY OF THE PINEAPPLE

The pineapple plant *(Ananas comosus)*, was found growing in a wild state along the sandy shores of tropical South America and the West Indies. It is neither a pine nor an apple, and its name is only an illustrative term for its form which resembles a pine cone. It is not even a fruit, but a *sorosis,* a multiple group of berries grown together into a pulpy mass from a spike of blossoms. The pineapple, whose name in Carib was *ananas,* was an important medicinal plant for the Indians. Its fermented juice was made into an alcoholic drink, used for fevers and to relieve body heat in hot weather; externally pineapple juice was used for dissolving painful corns, and to cure skin ailments. The greatest value of pineapple juice lies in its digestive power, which closely resembles that of human gastric juices. The Indians cooked and baked their meat overlaid with chunks of pineapple. This had a tenderizing effect on the toughest animal meat and was the culinary forerunner of our southern ham, decorated with pineapple slices. The pineapple was one of the tropical plants which for centuries resisted successful transplantation to other continents. Pineapples seemingly would not grow from seeds anywhere; they could only be raised from slips of the plant, which would not endure the slow and long sea-voyages of bygone centuries, rotting away and fermenting in the steaming holds of the sailing vessels. Only a few potted plants, carefully tended on their Atlantic crossing, reached European shores where they were kept in the hothouses of royal gardens as curious specimens of tropical flora. In the second half of the 19th century, when the invention of the

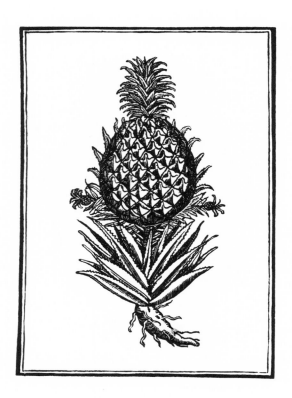

Pineapple, from Dalechamp's HISTORIA PLANTARUM,
Lyons, 1587.

THE STORY OF THE PINEAPPLE

screw-propeller driven steamboat shortened the shipping time of perishable cargo, the first West Indian pineapples were introduced into tropical Africa and reached the Malay Peninsula from there. At the end of the 19th century, Singapore was the world's main shipping port for cultivated pineapples. In 1899, the pineapple was introduced into Hawaii where the plant found ideal climatic conditions. The improvement in the preservation process at the beginning of the present century and the canning of ripe pineapples directly on the plantation greatly expanded the distribution of pineapples which are now grown not only in Brazil, Cuba, Puerto Rico, the Bahamas, Malaya, the Philippines, Hawaii and other tropical countries, but also in Mexico, Florida and other southern territories of North America; Singapore eventually lost its eminence to the Hawaiian Islands which today produce the lion's share of the world's pineapple crop. The fine, strong and flexible fiber obtained from the leaves of the pineapple is used in Brazil, Malaya and the Philippines in the manufacture of a native textile, delicate, soft, transparent piña-cloth from which luxurious scarves, handkerchiefs and embroidered fashion accessories are made. Today the pineapple in the form of fresh, canned or candied fruit is an important international trade item, and canned pineapple juice is used as a refreshing beverage in many parts of the world.

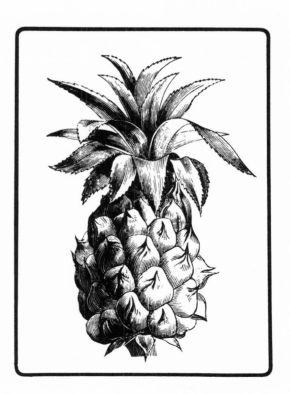

True Pineapple, from Strässle's NATURGESCHICHTE, *Stuttgart, 1885.*

THE STORY OF THE POMEGRANATE

Assyrian Banquet Food, from a wall carving in ancient Nineveh.

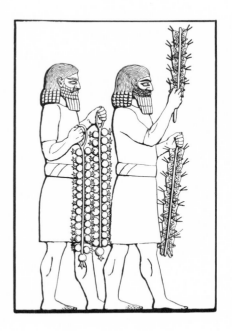

The many-seeded fruit of the pomegranate tree *(Punica granatum),* native to the Near East and tropical Africa, is one of the oldest Semitic symbols of life, fertility and abundance. The pomegranate, along with wheat and the grape, was regarded as one of the prime attributes of *Ibritz,* the Hittite god of agriculture. It was embroidered at the hem of Aaron's sacred robes and adorned the official vestments of the priest-kings of ancient Persia. The capitals and pillars of the Temple of Solomon were covered with carved pomegranates. Pomegranates were served at the marriage banquets of ancient Assyria and Babylonia as a symbol of love and fecundity. When the pomegranate traveled from Asia Minor to the Far East, its symbolic meaning

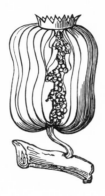

The Pomegranate Badge of Katherine of Aragon.

THE STORY OF THE POMEGRANATE

accompanied it. At Oriental weddings, seeds of the pomegranate were offered to the guests and, when the newly-weds entered their bedchamber, pomegranates were thrown to the floor and the bursting fruits strewed their seeds all over the room, signifying that the marriage should be happy and blessed with many children. When the Moors conquered Spain about 800 A.D., they introduced the pomegranate into the Iberian peninsula and the fruit became the emblem of Granada, whose name was derived from it. Catherine of Aragon (1485-1536), the first wife of Henry VIII, wore the Spanish emblem of the pomegranate, and the Oriental fruit became the badge of their daughter, Mary Tudor (1516-1558), Queen of England. The name of the pomegranate was derived from the Latin *pomum* — apple, and *granatum* — with seeds. When the explosive shell that strewed metal particles over a wide area was invented, the French, mindful of the seed-scattering characteristics of the pomegranate, called it *grenade*, and the special regiments, founded in 1791, who launched these new weapons, were called *grenadiers*. Presumably, the pomegranate was introduced into the new world by the early Spanish colonists and has since been commonly cultivated in gardens ranging from the warmer sections of the United States to Chile. Small commercial plantings have been made in California. Though pomegranates will grow in a wide range of climates, good fruit is produced only where high temperature and dry atmosphere accompany the ripening period. Varieties cultivated in the United States are the Wonderful, the Paper-Shell, and the Spanish Ruby.

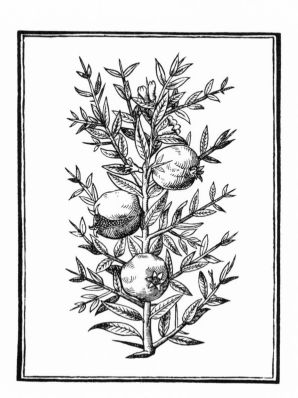

Pomegranate, from Mattioli's COMMENTAIRES, *Lyons, 1579.*

THE STORY OF THE POTATO

The potato plant *(Solanum tuberosum)* originated in the Andes region of South America, spreading gradually among the Indian tribes of the Americas. Its name came from the Haitian *batata,* changed to the Spanish *patata,* and finally to the English *potato.* One of Francisco Pizarro's priests introduced potatoes into Spain in 1534. Here they were hailed as a revitalizer for impotence, and were sold on the strength of that belief for fantastic prices, in some instances as high as one thousand dollars a pound. In 1565, Sir John Hawkins brought the potato plant to Ireland and, in 1585, Sir Francis Drake introduced it to England. Potatoes were reluctantly accepted as food in Europe because the population feared that they were poisonous. Ireland, a poor agricultural country, was the first to recognize the food value of the potato. In 1719, the first plants were carried from Ireland to the North American continent by a group of Presbyterian emigrants. In the meantime, in 1728, Scotland prohibited the cultivation of potatoes on the grounds that they were an unholy nightshade and not mentioned in the Bible. Baron Antoine-Augustin Parmentier, agriculturist and economist, introduced the potato into France in 1785, and boosted its use by devising numerous methods and recipes for its preparation. Thus the lowly potato finally became an esteemed, daily food item throughout the western world. According to the Irish proverb: *Be eating one potato, peeling a second, have a third in your fist, and your eye on a fourth.*

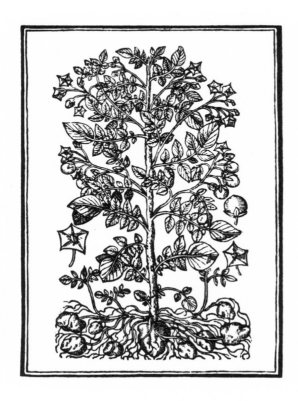

Potato Plant, from Bauhin's PRODROMOS, *Frankfort/M., 1620.*

THE STORY OF RUBBER

Rubber is mainly the product of the milky juice of two trees, the rubber tree *(Hevea brasiliensis),* native to the Amazon basin in South America, and the guttapercha tree *(Palaquium gutta),* originating in Borneo, Sumatra and the Malay Peninsula. The use of rubber by the Indians of Mexico was discovered by the Spanish in 1521. Gonzales Hernandez de Oviedo y Valdes in his *Historia General,* published in 1535, was the first to mention the Indian ball game of *Batey,* played with a ball, called *batos,* made of an unknown resilient substance. This material was the sap of the rubber tree, from which the Indians made not only balls, but also watertight shoes. They would dunk their feet a few times into the sap of these trees, let it dry, then peal off the made-to-order rubbers for further use. No one in Europe was interested in this material for the next 200 years, until, in 1736, the French physician and naturalist, M. de la Condamine, brought back from an expedition into Ecuador a sample of *caoutchouc* (from its Carib name *cahuchu*) to the French Academy of Science for the study of its unusual properties. In 1755, Don Jose of Portugal, who heard of the wonderful waterproof material used by the Indians, sent several pairs of his boots with a royal expedition to Para, Brazil, in order that they might be waterproofed with this gum. In 1762, it was discovered that the natives of Penang, Malaya, carried their water and food in vessels and bags made from the hardened latex of a native tree *(Ficus elastica)* in Malaya. In the year 1770, the English chemist, Joseph Priestley, found that a piece of this gum wiped the marks of black lead pencil from paper. This first use of the strange

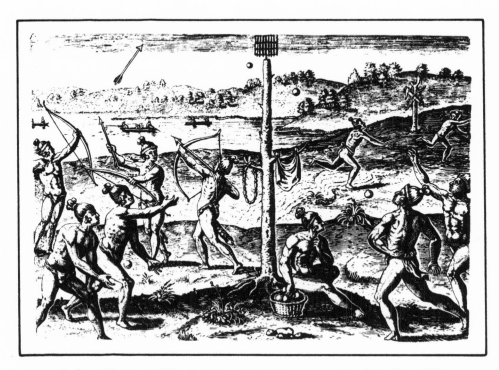

Indians Playing Rubber-ball, from de Bry's FLORIDA, *Frankfort/M., 1591.*

THE STORY OF RUBBER

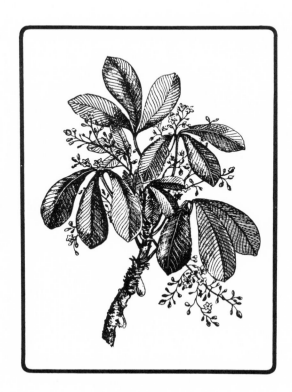

Pará Rubber Tree, from an old American engraving.

material for *rubbing* pencil lines from paper is responsible for the name *rubber* and, since it came from the faraway lands of the Indians, its official name became *India rubber*. A Scotsman from Glasgow, Charles Macintosh, invented the waterproofing process that applied rubber to fabrics in 1823. He established a factory in Manchester and became the father of the raincoat industry. In 1835, the first solid rubber tires for coaches were produced in France, to be used instead of the usual iron tires. The American inventor, Charles Goodyear, took out a patent for the vulcanizing process of rubber on February 24, 1839, but not much interest was shown in this new invention by American industrialists. In 1850, in Vienna, the Austrian manufacturer, Joseph Reithofer, founded a factory for making vulcanized rubber boots, the first important industrial item made from vulcanized rubber. The rising demand for rubber induced the British government to break the monopoly of Brazil on crude rubber. Since the Brazilian government had prohibited the taking out of a single hevea seed from that country, Englishmen tried time and again to smuggle seeds out of Brazil, risking their liberty, and even their lives, without success. In 1875, Benjamin Disraeli, Prime Minister of England, sent a botanical expedition under Henry A. Wickham of Kew Gardens to Brazil. Wickham went up the Amazon River in a little ocean-going steamer to collect specimens of exotic plants for the Botanical Gardens in London. After he had packed all his collected plants into open Indian baskets, he strewed them with 7000 hevea seeds and sailed boldly down the Amazon estuary with a

THE STORY OF RUBBER

declared cargo of *"exceedingly delicate botanical specimens"*. He passed with flying colors under the guns of the Brazilian customs men who could not imagine that anyone would be so brazen as to smuggle such a fantastic quantity of hevea seeds out in the open, before their watchful eyes. These thousands of seeds were planted in Kew Gardens and the young plants shipped to every corner of the British colonies for replanting. Today the vast rubber plantations in the Far East alone number more than a billion hevea trees. The greatest impetus to the rubber industry was the improved version of Thompson's pneumatic tire, patented on December 7, 1888, by the Scotch inventor, John Boyd Dunlop, whose tires made possible the rise of the bicycle industry and, later on, of its gargantuan offspring, the automobile industry. Rubber today has found hundreds of vital industrial uses. Recently it has been used in composite structures with other materials such as textiles, metals, wood, glass, asbestos and other components. The development of reinforcing pigments such as carbon blacks has imparted to cured rubber marked improvement in resistance to tear and abrasion. The fact that Japan controlled 90% of the world's supply of rubber in 1941, as a result of its empire expansion in World War II, made it imperative for western nations to mass-produce synthetic rubber. However, with the advance into the space age, still newer and more important uses for natural rubber have been created. Thus, rubber more than continues to hold its own as a leading basic material in our technological age.

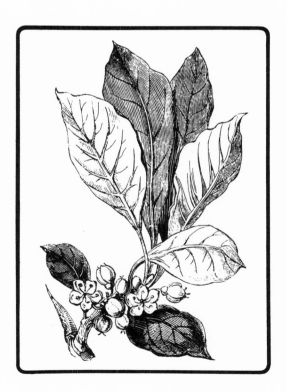

Gutta-percha Tree, from an old English engraving.

THE STORY OF SUGAR

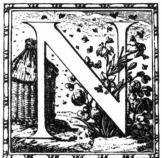

N O OTHER VEGETABLE PRODUCT is as old as sugar. Sugar in any form is not only a pleasant sweetening agent, but also one of the most important food items of the human race. Honey is the oldest natural sugar supply, known from the time the first prehistoric man observed a bear raiding the honey hoard of a wild bee swarm. He tried it too and loved it. Honey became so important to humanity that in order to have a steady supply at hand, man domesticated the bee which became the only insect that has the distinction of working full time for its human masters. In Greek mythology, the infant Zeus was hidden by his mother, Rhea, in a cave on Mount Ida, Crete, to shield the child from the wrath of his father, Cronus. Bees came along and fed him honey. For reward, Zeus endowed them with high intelligence. Meanwhile, in order that the hiding place not be betrayed by the cries of the child, relays of Cretan

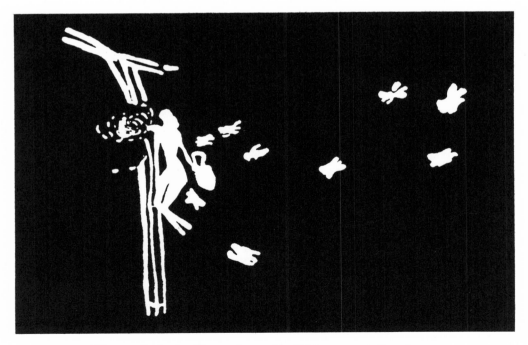

Woman Gathering Honey, from a Neolithic cave painting, Arana.

THE STORY OF SUGAR

priestesses of Rhea danced before the cave to the clash of swords, shields and cymbals. Since that time, bees were believed to be susceptible to the din of metallic percussion instruments. This gave rise to the apiarist's old custom of striking pans to *"ring in the bees"*, the din being expected to make the insects settle down. Sugar was still an expensive commodity, and so important was honey as a sweetening agent in 17th century England, that Moses Rusden, Beemaster to the King's most excellent Majesty, by royal command and at the expense of Charles II, published in 1685 at London a book *"A Full Discovery of Bees"*, to propagate more modern keeping methods for apiaries. Man's hunger for sugar led him to experiment with whatever sweet tasting plant he could unearth. We know of the grape and fruit sugars of antiquity; the East Indian *jaggery,* a coarse sugar produced from the sap of the sugar palm *(Arenga pinnata);* the sorghum syrup of the Far East and Africa, derived from the sweet sorghum grass *(Sorghum vulgare);* the birch sugar of Scandinavia and Scotland, condensed from the sap of the sweet birch *(Betula pubescens),* and the maple sugar of the North American Indians, produced from the sap of the sugar maple *(Acer saccharum);* the *agavose,* a sugar manufactured by the Mexican Indians from the stalks of the century plant *(Agave americana);* the raisin sugar of the Levant, the malt, corn syrup, potato sugar, and many, many more sugary and syrupy derivatives of plants, invented and used throughout the millennia by man in his craving and quest for sugar. But aside from honey, only cane sugar became of world wide importance, joined in our time by beet sugar. With the steadily growing production of cane and beet sugar in the agricultural

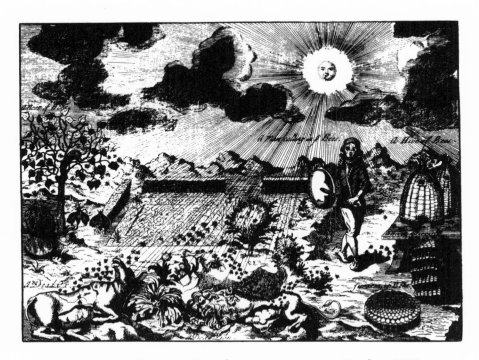

Ringing in the Bees, from Pomet's HISTORY OF DRUGGS, *London, 1725.*

THE STORY OF SUGAR

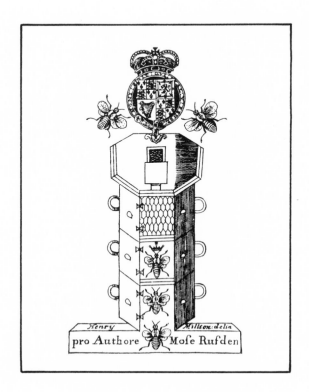

Frontispiece, from Rusden's A FULL DISCOVERY OF BEES, *London, 1685.*

production of many lands, sugar is today not only a food and a condiment, but also an important preservative for other food products. It also became one of the most widely used basic production materials in many gigantic industries of our time. Enormous quantities of sugar are consumed in the manufacture of alcoholic beverages, soft drinks and chocolates. The canning industry uses sugar as a main ingredient in canned fruits, jams, marmalades, jellies and evaporated milk, and as a condiment and preservative in canned soups, vegetables, and in hundreds of other food products. Cereal manufacturers use sugar as a sweetening agent, as do many other food industries. The meat packers use it for sugar cured ham, bacon and other meat products. Thus, one of the costliest foods of bygone days has changed its status to that of a fairly cheap and all important mainstay of our daily diet.

THE CANE SUGAR

The sugar cane *(Saccharum officinarum)*, a tall tropical grass native to India, was introduced to Persia at the end of the 3rd century A.D. by the Sassanid Caliphs, where it was successfully planted along the river-banks in the Susiana Province. It was introduced to Arabia in the 5th century A.D., and in the 9th century A.D., the Saracens brought the plant to Egypt where it was cultivated extensively in the Nile Delta. With the advance of the Moslem conquerors along

THE STORY OF SUGAR

the Mediterranean region, sugar cane was introduced to Cyprus, Sicily, Spain, Portugal, Madeira and the Canary Islands. In 1493, on his second voyage, Christopher Columbus carried seedlings of this plant from Gomera, one of the Canary Islands, to San Domingo. By 1518, Spanish settlers were operating 28 sugar plantations in San Domingo, from which came the bulk of the European sugar supply. In 1646, the British started to cultivate sugar cane in their oldest settlement in the Caribbean, Barbados. The product of the sugar cane changed its name with the changing nationality of the plant. Its original name in Indian Sanscrit was *sarcara,* modified to the Indian Prakrit *sakara,* changed on its journey to the Persian *shakar,* the Greek *sachar,* the Latin *succarum,* the Italian *zucchero,* the Spanish *azúcar,* the German *zucker,* the French *sucre,* and finally to the English *sugar.* Today sugar cane is cultivated in every tropical and semi-tropical country, not only in the Mediterranean region, from the Near East to the Canary Islands, but also in the West Indies from Cuba to Trinidad, on the mainland of North, Central and South America from Louisiana to Argentina, and in the Far East from Hawaii to the Malaccan Coast of the Malay Peninsula. Quite an achievement for one of today's staple foods! Sugar was so costly 500 years ago that in Europe only the very rich courtiers and dandies could afford it and they carried little lumps of plain or candied sugar in silver boxes, offering these rare and greatly coveted tidbits in oriental fashion, with an elegant flourish, to their

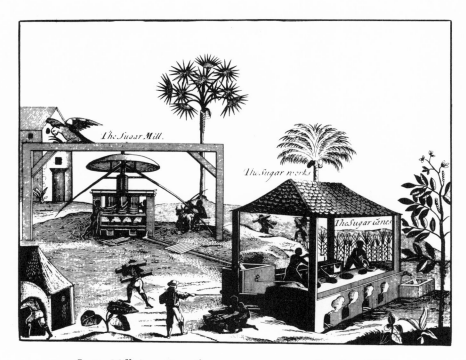

Sugar Mill, from Pomet's HISTORY OF DRUGGS, *London, 1725.*

THE STORY OF SUGAR

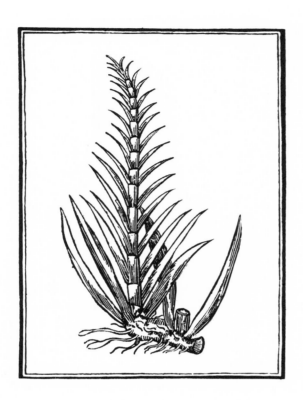

Sugar Cane, from Gerard's HERBALL, *London, 1633.*

ladies. These little lumps of plain sugar were the great-granddaddies of our sugar candy, and even our English name for it comes from the Indian Sanskrit *sarcara khanda* — a broken piece of sugar. One of the by-products of cane sugar refining in the West Indies is a dark colored molasses, from the Latin *mellaceus* — like honey, which is one of the basic ingredients for the distillation of rum. Freshly distilled rum is clear, like water, and the coloring is accomplished by adding caramel and by storage in old sherry casks.

THE SUGAR BEET

The sugar beet *(Beta vulgaris)* is a root plant whose large white or yellow root contains about 15% sugar. Native to western Asia and Europe, beets were known in antiquity and cultivated by the Greeks and Romans as far back as 300 B.C. For over 2000 years, the sugar beet was used only as a vegetable and a cattle feed because its sugar content could not be extracted from the root by any known method. In 1747, at Berlin, the German chemist, Andreas Sigismund Margraff, invented a process to extract the sugar from beets, but it took nearly 130 years to adapt his chemical method to a commercially sound production process, and to develop the necessary machinery. When new sugar-mill machines were finally exhibited in 1878 at the World's Fair in Paris, every European country from France to Russia became interested in

THE STORY OF SUGAR

cultivating its own beet crop and in manufacturing its own beet sugar to escape the heavy financial burden of cane sugar imports from overseas. The Congress of the United States called for a special report on the subject and, in 1880, the first sugar beets were planted in several states of the Union, encouraged by bounties to farmers from the federal government and various state legislatures. The planting of sugar beets in Europe and North America increased rapidly in the 1890's, and the national production of beet sugar in all the former sugar-importing countries expanded to such proportions that the commercial situation on the plantations in the cane-sugar producing West Indies and other tropical countries became desperate and verged closely on ruin. At the turn of the century the peoples of the western world consumed two pounds of beet sugar to each pound of cane sugar. The repeal of sugar bounties in all beet growing countries at the beginning of our century swung the pendulum back to a more even consumption. In the United States, as a result of the cruder methods for beet sugar production in the beginning, a certain prejudice against the product developed and still exists today. However, with modern improved refining methods for beet sugar, this popular sentiment has little basis because, in practice, the consumer can not tell the difference between properly refined cane or beet sugar. There is no difference in appearance, sweetness, flavor or composition, either by taste or by analysis.

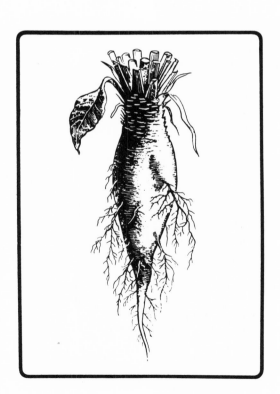

Sugar Beet, from Strässle's NATURGESCHICHTE, *Stuttgart, 1888*

THE STORY OF THE TOMATO

The tomato plant *(Lycopersicon esculentum)*, native to South America, was cultivated by the Incas, Mayas, Aztecs, and their predecessors since time immemorial. Its name is derived from the Aztec *tomatl*, transformed into the Spanish *tomate*, and finally into the English *tomato*. Shortly after the conquest of Mexico, seeds of the tomato plant were brought by a caravel to Spain and planted in Morocco, across the Straits of Gibraltar. From there the plant reached Italy, where it was called *pomo dei mori* — apple of the Moors (later changed to *pomo d'ore* — golden apple). It was introduced to France as an aphrodisiac, and the French misspelled its name as *pomme d'amour* — apple of love. In Germany it was called *paradies apfel* — apple of Paradise, because it was believed that the Turks brought it from the Holy Land, the original location of the Biblical Paradise. The tomato reached England under the name *pome amoris* — love-apple, and later, under that name, was carried back over the Atlantic by colonists to the American continent. In all its extended travels, the tomato was never used as food. It was not eaten by the Europeans, because, as a relative of the deadly nightshade, it was considered poisonous and was grown only as a decorative garden shrub. This superstition vanished suddenly at the beginning of the 19th century in North America and the tomato became, around 1830, an important food crop for the American market. Contrary to a widespread belief, the tomato is neither a vegetable nor a fruit, but, botanically, is considered a berry.

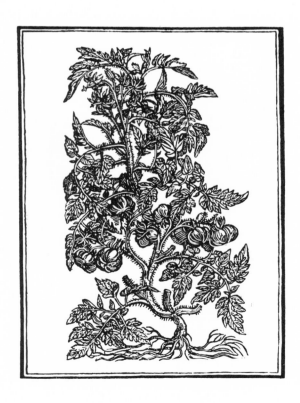

Apples of Love, from Gerard's HERBALL, *London, 1633.*

THE PHYSIC GARDEN

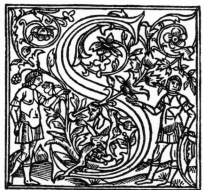

INCE EARLY TIMES plants have provided the medicinal remedies of the human race. The whole structure of modern pharmacopeia is based on man's historical knowledge of flowers, herbs, plants and trees. Nature has provided a complete storehouse of herbal remedies to cure all ills of mankind, and today's medicines are only the chemical-pharmaceutical translations of the healing properties of herbs. Looking back through history, we find there is not a single plant that has not been used at one time or another by men as a foodstuff, a healing, life-giving medicine, or a deadly poison. Since the dawn of civilization man has fed on berries, fruits, grasses, herbs, leaves and roots. His selection of vegetable food in these prehistoric times was entirely by trial and error. He continued to eat the plants that agreed with him while remaining away from those that made him ill. After man mastered the use of fire, the roasted flesh of animals came into the foreground of the human diet and he began the domestication of animals for his daily needs. The shepherds of the tribal community flocks, remaining close to nature and having plenty of time during their lonely tasks, observed the behavior of various plants and the effects on their animal charges. In this way they became the sages and medicine men of their tribes. These herb-wise shepherds and medicine men of prehistoric times developed into the herbalists of ancient Persia and the philosophers of

THE STORY OF HERBS

antiquity. In addition to their necessary food-plants, all the old agricultural nations cultivated herbs for their medicinal needs. In the early days of the Christian Church, the cultivation of herbs was forbidden. Knowledge of herbs was considered pagan because of the many mystic and magical rites connected with their use. In the Dark Ages many of the herbal manuscripts of early days were destroyed by the martial rulers and their mercenaries who were devoid of any interest in science and culture. The knowledge of herbs and their properties was kept alive only by the monks in the seclusion and comparative security of their monasteries. They studied, translated and copied painstakingly by hand again and again, the few remaining herbals for posterity. In the later Middle Ages the cultivation of herbs was again taken up by monks and nuns, who were not only healers of the soul, but also physicians and nurses to their

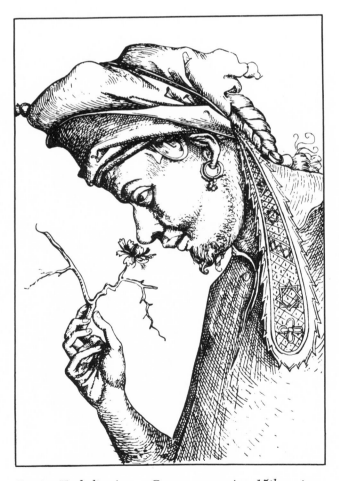

Persian Herbalist, from a German engraving, 15th century.

THE STORY OF HERBS

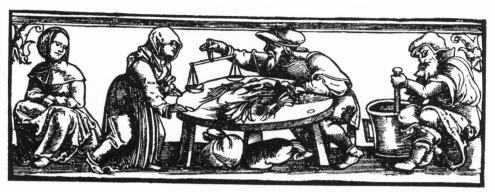

Herbman, from Friess' SPIEGEL DER ARTZNEY, *Strasbourg, 1529.*

flocks. The herb garden, called *Physick Garden*, became part and parcel of every cloister and monastery and, later on, of every castle, court, hospital and medical college. Alembic laboratories, or distilling plants, the nuclei of our modern pharmaceutical industry, were set up in monasteries and hospitals to convert the herb crop into medical potions and liquors. The rise of the chemical-pharmaceutical industry made the bulk of these herbal concoctions obsolete,

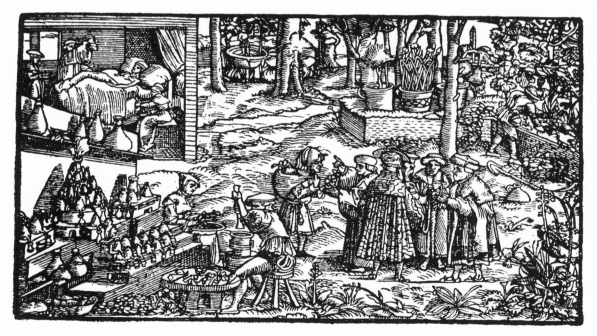

Physic Garden, from Petrarca's TROSTSPIEGEL, *Augsburg, 1531.*

THE STORY OF HERBS

but we still use many as spices and condiments for our food, in medicinal teas and infusions, and monastery herb liquors such as Benedictine, Peres Chartreuse, Trappistine, and others continue to serve as stomachic tonics. Throughout human history, flowers, plants, trees and herbs became so interwoven with man's daily life that they developed into symbols for his expressions and sentiments, passions and affections, fears and superstitions. In ancient

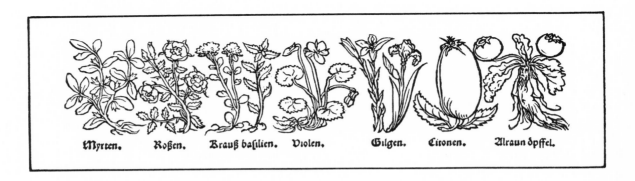

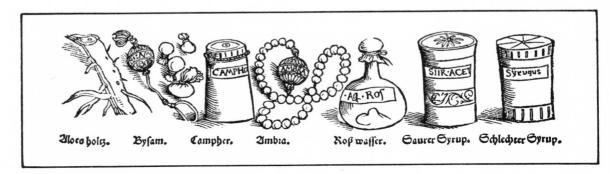

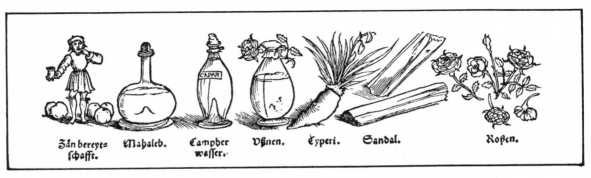

Medicaments, from Hero's SCHACHTAFELN DER GESUNTHEYT, *Strasbourg, 1533.*

THE STORY OF HERBS

mythology, folklore and legend, the fertile human mind assigned to plants their medicinal and nutritive properties. The religious, legendary and symbolic meaning attached to plants has been handed down to us through the ages and today we still use many special plants in accordance with their age-old symbolism, as at Easter, Christmas, St. Patrick's and numerous other holidays and special occasions.

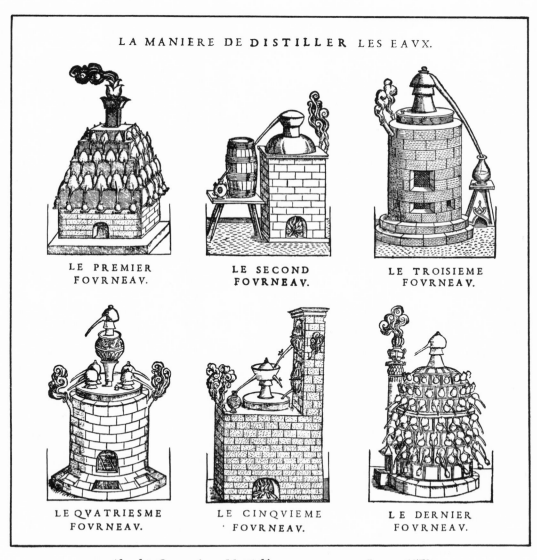

LA MANIERE DE **DISTILLER** LES EAVX.

LE PREMIER FOVRNEAV.

LE SECOND FOVRNEAV.

LE TROISIEME FOVRNEAV.

LE QVATRIESME FOVRNEAV.

LE CINQVIEME FOVRNEAV.

LE DERNIER FOVRNEAV.

Alembic Ovens, from Mattioli's COMMENTAIRES, *Lyons, 1579.*

THE ABSINTH

The absinth or wormwood plant *(Artemisia absinthium)*, native to Europe, is now grown all over the world from the United States to Siberia. The absinth liqueur, distilled from the dark green oil of this plant and anise, was more intoxicating than any other liqueur. Habitual drinking of too much absinth causes absinthism, a diseased condition which can lead to complete paralysis. At the beginning of World War I, excessive consumption of absinth caused so many deaths in France that the French government was forced to prohibit its manufacture in 1915. Wormwood is used today only for flavoring tonics, vermouth wines and stomachic liquors.

Absinth, from Mattioli's COMMENTAIRES, *Lyons, 1579.*

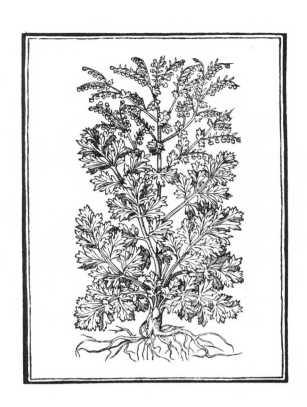

THE BELLADONNA

Belladonna *(Atropa belladonna)* is the deadly nightshade plant, native to Europe, whose drug property is the poisonous atropin. Its name was derived from the Italian *bella* — beautiful, and *donna* — lady. The plant got this name in the time of the Italian Renaissance, the days of the Borgias, when poison was so popular that poison rings, stilettos and pellets were kept around the palace, just in case. The ladies of the court used one of these poisons, belladonna, not to kill their rivals, but to beautify and enlarge the pupils of their eyes. Atropin is still used in modern medicine to stimulate the heart, relieve spasms and expand the pupils of the eye during ophthalmologic examination.

Belladonna, from Mattioli's COMMENTAIRES, *Lyons, 1579.*

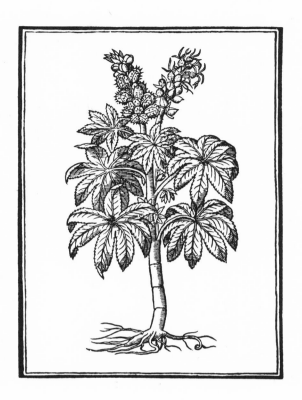

THE CASTOR OIL PLANT

The castor oil plant *(Ricinus communis)*, also called *palma Christi,* native to western Asia and Africa, bears bean-like seeds. These are the castor beans from which castor oil has been pressed since antiquity. It is one of the oldest medicinal prescriptions, used throughout the ages as a purgative for all ills of the stomach, spleen, bowels, uterus, and as a cure for intestinal worms. A concoction of its roots was used to relieve kidney and bladder troubles; and an infusion of its leaves as a remedy for scabby, rash, itch and inflammation of the eye. Castor oil is still used today as a purgative for constipation and tapeworms, much to the displeasure of both children and adults.

Castor Oil Plant, from Mattioli's COMMENTAIRES, *Lyons, 1579.*

THE GARLIC

The garlic plant *(Allium sativum),* a member of the lily family, has been used since early antiquity in the Orient and Occident as an antiseptic protection against the plague, a potent medicinal remedy for all diseases of man and beast, a powerful charm against the evil eye, demons, witches, and vampires. In ancient Rome the garlic was dedicated to Mars, the god of war. The Roman legions propagated the garlic in all their conquered lands because it was believed that eating it in abundance gave courage on the battlefield. The English name of the garlic is derived from the Old English *gar* — spear, and *leac* — leek.

Garlic, from Mattioli's COMMENTAIRES, *Lyons, 1579.*

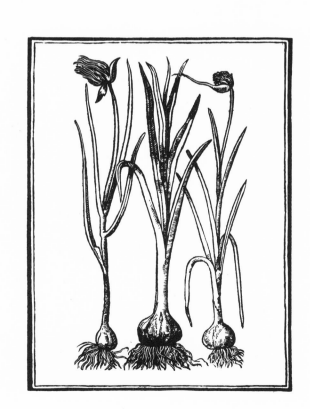

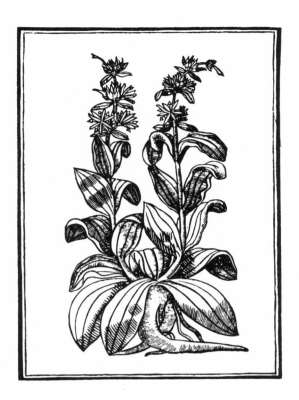

THE GENTIAN

The gentian plant *(Gentiana lutea)* was named after Gentius, King of Illyria (180 B.C.), who was supposed to be the first to discover the medicinal virtues of this herb. Throughout the centuries, the bitter juice of the gentian root has been used as a stomach tonic, an antidote against the poisonous bite of mad dogs and venomous reptiles, a remedy for diseases of the stomach and the liver, a powerful cure for the plague. Its leaves, steeped in wine, were taken to provide refreshment for fatigue and as a warming tonic for exposure. Today, the juice of the gentian root is still an important ingredient in stomach-bitters prescribed to aid digestion and to remedy stomach aches.

Gentian, from Mattioli's COMMENTAIRES, *Lyons, 1579.*

THE GINSENG

The ginseng *(Panax quinquefolius)* is an herb with a forked root, native to China and North America. In the Far East, the juice of this aromatic root is considered the ultimate elixir of life and a cure for all the ills of mankind. The plant itself is a Chinese symbol of strength, vigor, long life and clear judgment. Ginseng root juice is used in Japan as a potent tonic and prolonger of life; in India, as a cure for malaria. The ginseng crop on the North American continent has little or no domestic usefulness, but for years has been one of the most important American exports to China and other countries of the Far East. In the United States ginseng is used only as a demulcent in a few skin ointments.

Ginseng, from Barton's MEDICAL BOTANY, *Philadelphia, 1818.*

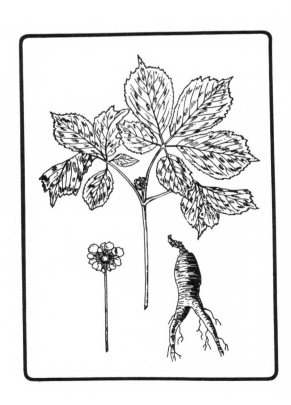

THE HEMLOCK

The poison hemlock *(Conium maculatum),* whose roots are deadly to humans but harmless to domesticated animals, is native to the Mediterranean region. It was the juice extracted from its roots that filled the notorious hemlock cup of ancient Athens, and of which the Greek philosopher, Socrates, drank and died. In medieval times, hemlock juice, added at the rate of one drop a day to a piece of sweet pastry, was used as a preventive against cholera, a remedy for hernia, epilepsy and pleurisy, and as a medicine for fainting spells and double vision. Today's *conium,* a powerful narcotic sedative, is derived from the dried, unripe fruit of the poison hemlock.

Hemlock, from Strässle's NATURGESCHICHTE, *Stuttgart, 1885.*

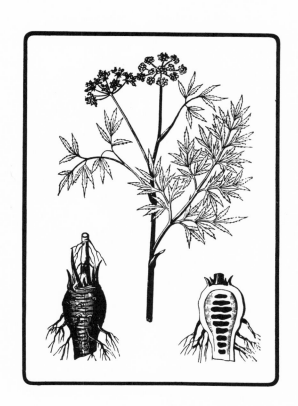

THE HENBANE

One of the most deadly members of the nightshade family, the henbane *(Hyoscyamus niger),* native to Europe, is a small herb with a hairy, sticky stem and a nauseating odor. Its name is derived from the Anglo-Saxon *henn*—chicken, and *bana*—murderer, because when fowls eat the seeds of this plant, they become paralyzed and die. These seeds are also poisonous to children, as well as rodents, pigs and fish. Nonetheless, because of its paralyzing effect, henbane juice in small quantities has been used as an antispasmodic for various conditions of asthma and whooping cough. Infusions of henbane have also been used as a mouthwash for toothache and as drops for earache.

Henbane, from Fuchs' DE HISTORIA STIRPIUM, *Basle, 1542.*

THE MUSTARD

The mustard plant *(Brassica nigra),* native to Asia, has been invading man's grainfields wherever he has begun to cultivate. Since antiquity, its pungent seeds have been used as a medicine by physicians. Mustard is one of the Biblical herbs. The ancient Greeks attributed its discovery to Asclepius. Its English name is derived from the fact that ground mustard seeds, mixed with *must,* were used as a condiment. Mustard seeds were chewed for toothache, taken internally for epilepsy, lethargy, stomach ache and for clarifying the blood. They were ground and sniffed to purge the brain by sneezing; externally, they were used as a poultice for pains and swellings and to draw splinters.

Mustard, from Mattioli's COMMENTAIRES, *Lyons, 1579.*

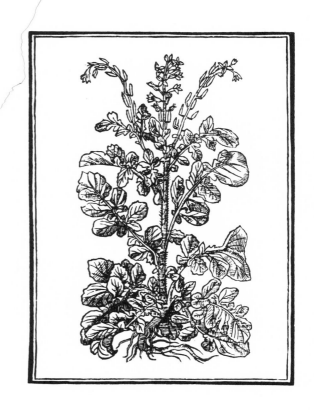

THE NETTLE

The stinging nettle *(Urtica dioica),* native to the Mediterranean region, was propagated by the Roman legions in their conquests all over Central Europe and into England. The Roman soldiers planted nettles, which are rich in formic acid, in every country where they found the climate cold. The soldiers, who could not stand the wet and chill of these regions, used to rub their limbs with the stinging nettles to warm their blood. In medieval times the juice, pressed from the whole plant, was used as medicine for tuberculosis. An infusion of the leaves served to relieve rheumatism and toothache, and the seeds were used as a remedy for dysentery. Nettle sprouts were eaten as a health salad.

Nettle, from Mattioli's COMMENTAIRES, *Lyons, 1579*

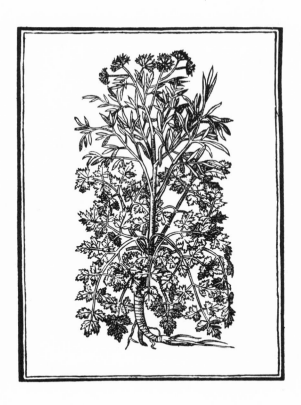

THE PARSLEY

The parsley *(Petroselinum crispum)*, native to North and Central Europe, enjoyed its greatest reputation among the ancient Greeks. At their banquets, they crowned their brows with its tendrils, believing that parsley not only created gaiety, but also increased the appetite. In the Dark Ages, it was believed that to transplant parsley was to invite death and crop failure. This superstition had its origin in the Roman custom of linking graves with parsley. In later medieval times, parsley was used for flatulence, stomach ache, cough and snake bite. An infusion of the young leaves was used as an eyewash; and a concoction of crushed seeds for freckles, as well as for head and body lice.

Parsley, from Mattioli's COMMENTAIRES, *Lyons, 1579.*

THE PEONY

As an infant, Asclepius, the son of Apollo, was entrusted to the care of Chiron, the wisest of the Centaurs, who instructed the boy in the art of healing. When Asclepius grew up he became the physician of the gods, and because of his medical knowledge was called *paeon* — helper. When Pluto was wounded by Hercules, Asclepius received from his grandmother, Leto, the goddess of darkness, a plant with which to cure Pluto. In Asclepius' honor, the plant was called peony *(Paeonia officinalis)*. From Greek antiquity to the Middle Ages the roots and seeds of the peony were considered among the most potent herbal cure-alls.

Peony, from Schöffer's HORTUS SANITATIS, *Mainz, 1485.*

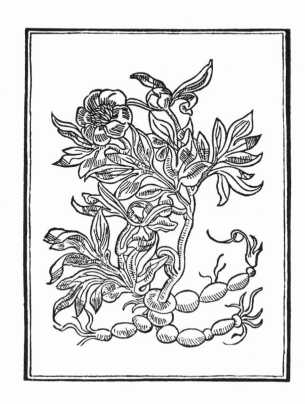

THE POPPY

The red or corn poppy *(Papaver rhoeas)* and the garden or opium poppy *(Papaver somniferum)*, both native to Eurasia, have been grown in the Near East since ancient times. The botanical name of the opium poppy is derived from Somnus, the Roman god of sleep, because the garden poppy is the source of one of the most powerful sleep-inducing narcotic drugs, opium, whose name is derived from the Greek *opion* — poppy juice. Morphine, an opium derivative, is named after Morpheus, the Greek god of dreams. Heroin, which is the German trade-name for a morphine derivative, was introduced to the medical world in 1898. The root of the poppy was used in ancient Assyria and Babylonia as an aphrodisiac. The juice of poppy seeds was well known to the ancient Egyptians as a sleep and dream inducing narcotic. The ancient Greeks used poppy seeds to relieve pain and procure sleep. The Greeks, who regarded sleep as the greatest of all physicians and the most powerful consoler of humanity, crowned all their nocturnal gods with a wreath of poppy blossoms. In Greek mythology the poppy was dedicated to Nix, goddess of night; to Thanatos, god of death; to his twin-brother Hypnos, god of sleep; and to the son of Hypnos, Morpheus, god of dreams. On this account, ever since antiquity, the poppy has been the symbol of consolation and oblivion. The opiate properties of poppy juice were mentioned by the Geek poet, Homer, as earuly as 850 B.C., and the use of poppy juice for medical purposes in the form of opium wine has been noted in the writings

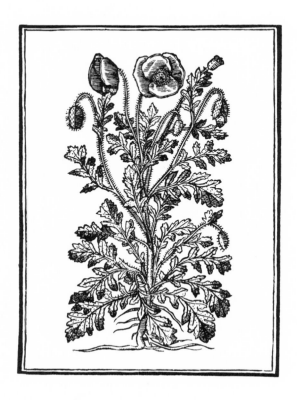

Corn Poppy, from Mattioli's COMMENTAIRES, *Lyons, 1579.*

THE POPPY

of the father of medicine, Hippocrates, the Greek physician (460-377 B.C.). The cultivation of the opium poppy spread with the march of Islam into Persia, Malaya and India. For centuries, poppies have been cultivated and opium manufactured in Bengal, the world's principal production center of the narcotic. The common notion that opium is typically Chinese is altogether false. Poppies were grown in Chinese gardens, but only as ornamental flowers, and not to provide a source of opium. The truth is that in the past century the East India Company, wishing to dispose of large quantities of opium manufactured in Bengal, sought to do so in China. This was opposed by the Chinese government, since the use of opium was forbidden in the Kingdom of the Middle. In the so-called Opium War that ensued (1839-1842), the drug was forced on China in unlimited quantities by the East India Company, aided by British and Oriental bootleggers who ran opium ships into Canton. Thus, the outlawed *Foreign Black Mud* was distributed in true gangster fashion all over the Chinese mainland, eventually destroying the power of the Chinese population to resist the commercial demands of the Western Powers. Opium was not manufactured in China proper before 1853. During 1931-1937, the Japanese, taking a leaf from history, ran another opium derivative, heroin, into China through Korea. They aimed at breaking the Chinese will to resist their domination. Today the three medically important and benevolent substances derived from the poppy —

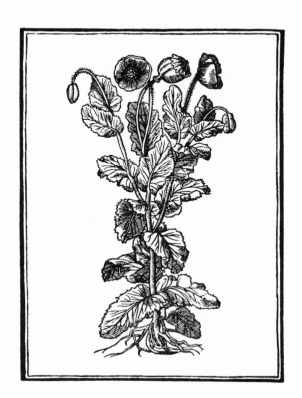

Garden Poppy, from Mattioli's COMMENTAIRES, *Lyons, 1579.*

THE POPPY

The Goddess of the Night, from an antique cameo.

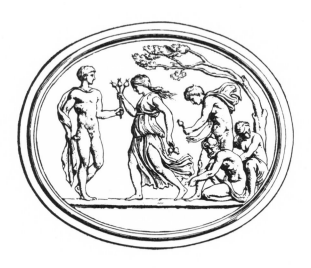

opium, morphine and heroin — have at the same time become the curse of humanity. They are smoked, eaten, drunk, sniffed or injected by untold millions of unfortunate addicts of all creeds and nationalities throughout the world. The distribution practices of present day narcotic rings are nothing new. They are only the modern continuation of the unsavory commercial practices of the China traders of 120 years ago. In antiquity the seeds of the corn poppy, which grew wild in the grain fields of the Near East, naturally got mixed in among the cereal seeds. Thus when these cereal seeds from the east were brought to western Europe and the British Isles, the poppy came along with them and spread through every land from east to west. One of the enjoyable products of the poppy is the poppy-seed which, for generations, has been used as a condiment in bread, pastry and other baked goods. The condiment is from either the black or white poppy, both of which are seed-heavy varieties of the opium poppy. Their seeds are so tiny that one pod may contain as many as thirty thousand of them. An old English custom to induce sleep in small children was to mix crushed poppy-seeds with their *pap,* made from bread boiled and softened in milk. The red corn poppy, considered the emblem of eternal sleep and oblivion, was believed to spring up on every battle-ground where men fought and died, deriving its red color from the blood of slain warriors. For centuries, the red poppy has been a symbol of fallen heroes in every war and, after World War I, the *poppies of Flanders* were adopted as the emblem of the U.S. Armistice Day, in memory of the dead of America's armed forces.

> "In Flanders' fields the poppies blow
> Between the crosses, row on row,
> That mark our place, and in the sky,
> The larks, still bravely singing, fly
> Scarce heard among the guns below."
>
> — *John McCrae*
> "Punch", December 8, 1915

THE SAGE

An evergreen plant of the mint family, the sage *(Salvia officinalis),* native to southern Europe and one of the most important medicinal herbs of antiquity, was dedicated to the Greek *Zeus,* and the Roman *Jupiter.* Its botanical name is derived from the Latin *salvus* — safe, so called for its reputed healing power. Throughout medieval Europe and England, long before the importation of Chinese tea, a tea made from sage was a daily beverage, not only because when sweetened with honey and mixed with milk it was a pleasant stimulant, but also because it was believed that a daily intake of sage was a panacea for many complaints. Accordingly, there is the old medieval proverb: *Why should a man die whilst sage grows in his garden.* Sage was one of the chief medicinal herbs of the Middle Ages; taken internally it was considered good for the liver, for breeding new blood in the body, the best food for the brain, an excellent strengthener of the muscles, and a tonic for stomach, heart and nerves. It was used as a remedy for ague, epilepsy, palsies, fevers and as a protection against the plague. An infusion of sage taken as a gargle was used to whiten the teeth and strengthen the gums. It was also considered a remedy for laryngitis, and in the form of antiseptic washes and compresses, was applied to bruises and sprains. Sage tea is still used today as an old-fashioned gargle and stomach tonic. Sage is also used extensively as a kitchen herb for flavoring soups and sauces and as a condiment for sausages and other meat products. A well known cheddar cheese, called *sage cheese,* is made by mixing green sage leaves into the curd before pressing.

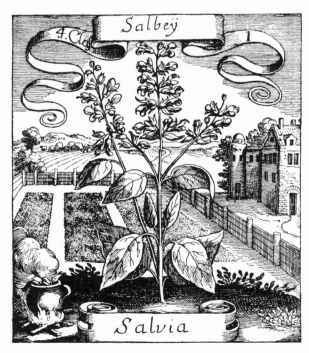

Sage, from Valentin's KRÄUTERBUCH, *Frankfort/M., 1719.*

THE SASSAFRAS

In 1586 when Sir Francis Drake brought the roots of the sassafras plant *(Sassafras albidum)* from North America to England, sassafras tea immediately gained wide favor as a cure-all. This tea, called *saloop*, was served in many little street stalls to English gentlemen who gathered to partake publicly of the remarkable new health brew. Spanish and French mercenaries, returning from the Americas, brought into Europe a new venereal disease, syphilis, which, it was then supposed, had been contracted from the Indians. When word reached England from the continent that sassafras tea was in reality the Indian cure for this so-called *French Pox*, the public drinking of *saloop* lost popularity.

Sassafras, from Monardes' JOYFULL NEWES, London, 1577.

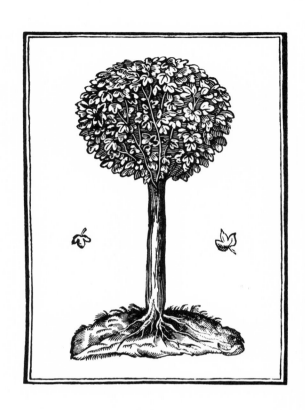

THE SESAME

The plant of *Open Sesame* fame was not only considered a magic plant, which could open caves and hidden passages, but also an important medicinal herb from the Orient. The seed of the sesame plant *(Sesamum indicum)*, native to Asia Minor and tropical regions, soaked in sparrow eggs and cooked in milk, was used for centuries as an aphrodisiac; sesame oil was applied externally as a cosmetic; it was mixed with vinegar as an ointment for the forehead to strengthen the brain, and blended with crow's gall as an embrocation for impotence. Today the oil of the sesame seed is one of the most important sources of fat in the Near and Far East.

Sesame, from Mattioli's COMMENTAIRES, Lyons, 1579.

THE CONFECTION BOX

In the 15th and 16th centuries, confect, or comfit was used as a household medicine, and the confection box played the part that our medicine cabinet plays today. A well stocked confection box contained twelve different kinds of sugary pastilles made from seeds, spices, and herbs mixed with honey and saffron. The usual ingredients of these pills were:

Almonds	Cinnamon	Fennel
Anise	Cloves	Ginger
Caraway	Coriander	Nutmeg
Cherry Kernels	Cubebs	Pepper

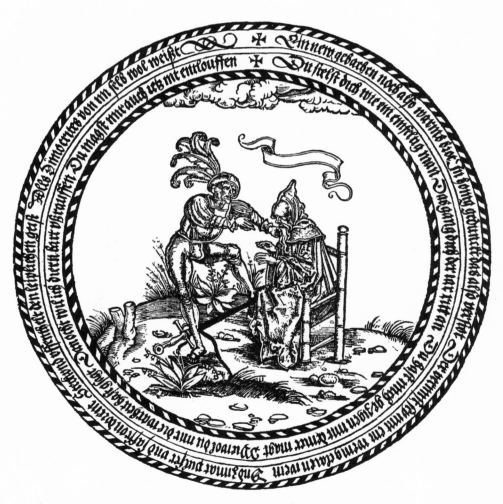

Decorative Lid from a Confection Box, Germany, 16th century.

THE CONFECTION BOX

THE ALMOND

The fruit of the almond tree *(Prunus amygdalis)*, native to Persia, was used as a remedy for insomnia and dysentery; an antidote for the influence of witch-craft and the evil eye, it served to stimulate the milk supply of nursing mothers, and to relieve headaches and hangover. Five almonds taken before drinking alcoholic beverages were considered the best bracer against intoxication and a preventive for hangovers.

Almonds, from Mattioli's COMMENTAIRES, *Lyons, 1579.*

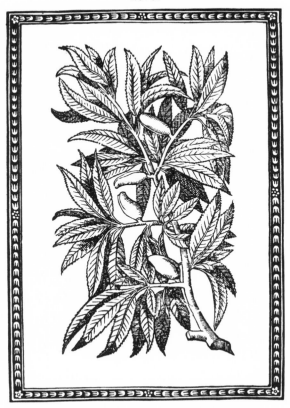

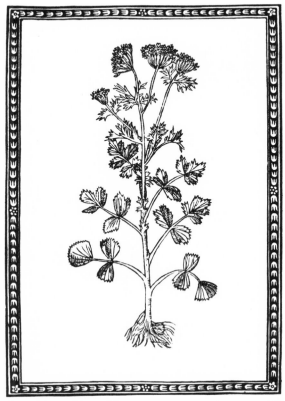

Anise, from Mattioli's COMMENTAIRES, *Lyons, 1579.*

THE ANISE

The dried seeds of the anise plant *(Pimpinella anisum)*, native to the Mediterranean region, an herb of the carrot family, were used as a purging agent for milt, kidneys, liver and gall; they served to relieve flatulence and were considered a remedy for worms, lice, scorbut, stomach-ache, vertigo, giddiness and nausea. They were also used to help increase the milk supply of nursing mothers and wet nurses.

THE CONFECTION BOX

THE CHERRY KERNELS

Cherry stones are the seeds of the cherry tree *(Prunus cerasus)*, native to Eurasia. Its kernels contain a volatile poison called prussic acid. This was used in small doses as a sedative for irritation of the throat and windpipe, to relieve chest pains, stomach and intestinal spasms, and as an anti-spasmodic for convulsions and the labor pain of expectant mothers. Six cherry kernels a day prevented the formation of kidney stones.

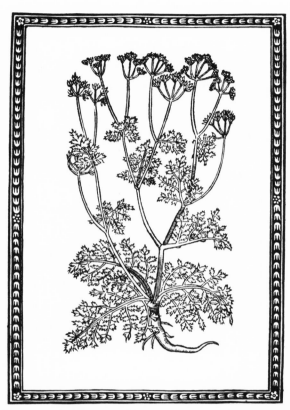

Caraway, from Mattioli's COMMENTAIRES, *Lyons, 1579.*

Cherries, from Mattioli's COMMENTAIRES, *Lyons, 1579.*

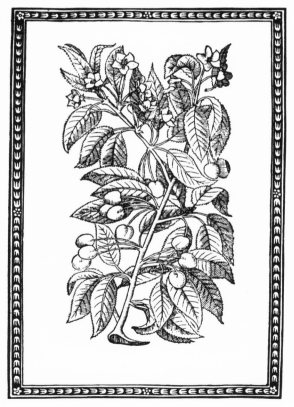

THE CARAWAY

The seed-like fruits of the caraway plant (*Carum carvi*), native to Europe, were used as a tonic to warm the stomach, to relieve flatulence, coughs, headaches, colic and frenzy, and as a potent antidote against the bite and sting of poisonous animals and insects. It was also believed that caraway seeds were a sure protection against loss of hair. Oil of caraway and sugar in alcohol was used to help relieve labor pains.

THE CONFECTION BOX

THE CINNAMON

The ground bark of the East Indian cinnamon tree *(Cinnamomum zeylanicum)*, native to Ceylon, India and Malaya, one of the oldest trade items from the Far East, has been used since antiquity as a breath sweetener, a tonic for the whole system: heart, stomach, liver, kidneys, gall and nerves. It was also considered a remedy for heartburn, nausea and diarrhoea, and as a sedative for expectant mothers during childbirth.

Cinnamon, from Jacobus' NEUW KREUTERBUCH, *Frankfort/M., 1613.*

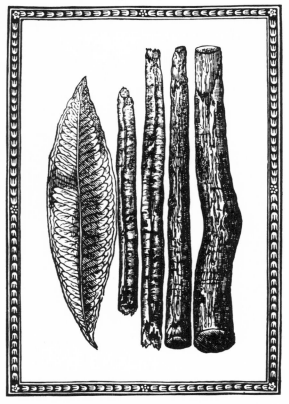

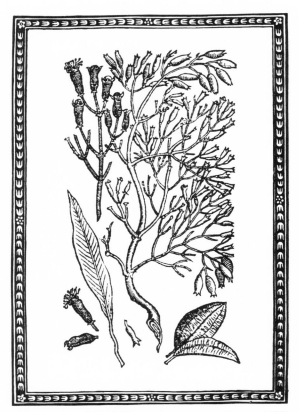

Cloves, from Mattioli's COMMENTAIRES, *Lyons, 1579.*

THE CLOVES

The dried, aromatic, immature flower-buds of the evergreen clove tree *(Syzygium aromaticum)*, native to the Molucca Islands, have been used since early times as a breath sweetener; a comforter for heart, liver, stomach and bowels; a remedy for nausea, colic, flatulence and diarrhoea; a preventive for paralysis of the tongue, inflammation of the gums, and loosening of the teeth. Rose water flavored with cloves was a favorite eyewash.

THE CONFECTION BOX

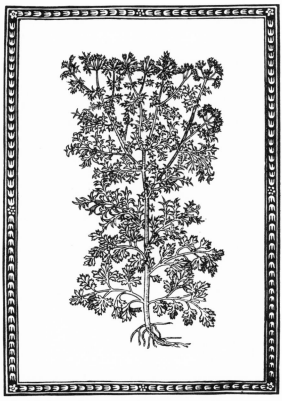

Coriander, from Mattioli's COMMENTAIRES, *Lyons, 1579.*

THE CUBEBS

The dried, unripe berries of the East Indian cubeb shrub *(Piper cubeba)*, native to the East Indies and the Malabar Coast, resemble the grains of black pepper but are less spicy and pungent. They were used extensively as a tonic for nerves and stomach, an abortive for kidney and bladder stones, a relief for epilepsy, asthma and other bronchial troubles, and as a potent laxative. Cubeb brandy was used to prevent venereal disease.

Cubebs, from Pomet's HISTORY OF DRUGGS, *London, 1725.*

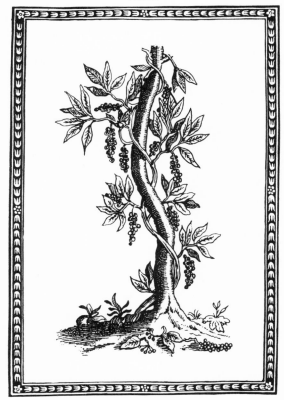

THE CORIANDER

The seed-like fruits of the coriander plant *(Coriandrum sativum)*, native to southern Europe, have been used since Biblical times by Egyptians and Hebrews as a purging agent for flatulence, constipation and delayed menstruation; a preventive against intermittent and puerperal fever, apoplexy and palsy. Sugar-coated coriander comfits were once highly prized as an aphrodisiac. Meat was preserved in coriander vinegar.

THE CONFECTION BOX

THE FENNEL

The dried seeds of the fennel plant *(Foeniculum vulgare)*, native to southern Europe, were used against mistiness of the eye and to drive worms out of the ears; to reduce excess flesh and fat; to relieve pains in the chest; to increase the milk supply of nursing mothers and as a general cleaning agent for the milt, liver, gall, kidneys and bladder. A solution of oil of fennel was used as an enema for hemorrhoids.

Fennel, from Mattioli's COMMENTAIRES, *Lyons, 1579.*

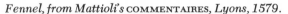

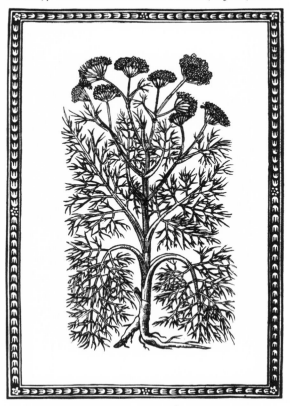

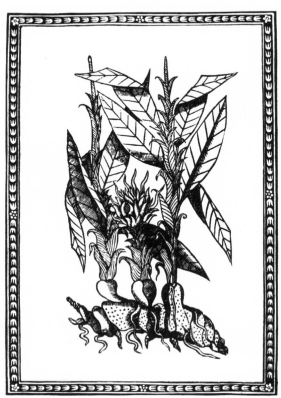

Ginger, from Acosta's TRACTADO DE LAS DROGAS, *Burgos, 1578.*

THE GINGER

The roots of the ginger reed plant *(Zingiber officinale)*, native to the Pacific Islands, were one of the important trade items of the Far East since antiquity. Raw and crystalized ginger was used as a breath sweetener, an aid to digestion and a relief for flatulence; a cure for toothache and bleeding gums and as a strengthening agent for loose teeth and weak eyes. A decoction of ginger and caraway in wine was used as a potent stomachic.

THE CONFECTION BOX

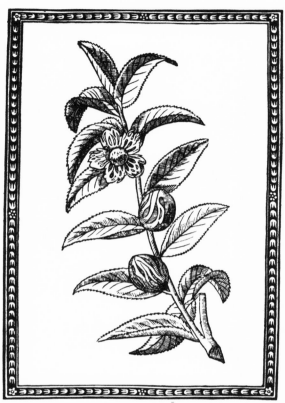

Nutmeg, from Mattioli's COMMENTAIRES, *Lyons, 1579.*

THE PEPPER

If ever there has been a cure-all remedy in popular medicine, it is the dried berry of the pepper tree *(Piper nigrum)*, native to the eastern tropics. It is the oldest trade item from the Orient. It has been used not only as a cure for everything from toothache to catalepsy, but also as a preventive drug for bloody dysentery, scarlet fever, smallpox, leprosy, typhus, cholera and the bubonic plague or the Black Death.

Pepper, from Acosta's TRACTADO DE LAS DROGAS, *Burgos, 1578.*

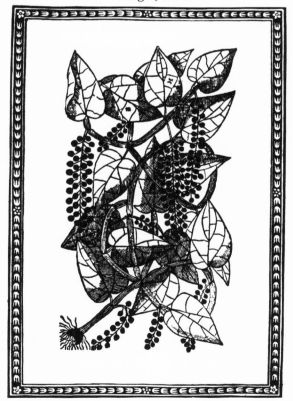

THE NUTMEG

The hard, aromatic fruit kernels of the East Indian nutmeg tree *(Myristica fragrans)*, native to the Molucca or Spice Islands, have been another important trade item of the Orient since antiquity. Because of their resemblance in shape to the human brain, nutmeg kernels were used as a remedy for all ailments of the brain, a cure for failing eyesight, and a general tonic and stimulant. Oil of nutmeg was used as an opiate.

THE CONFECTION BOX

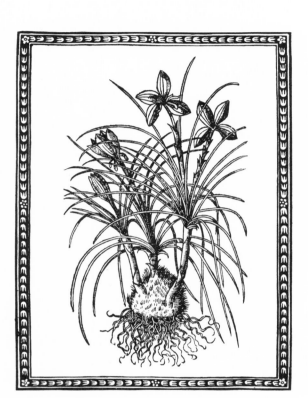

THE SAFFRON

The orange çolored, aromatic, pungent stigmas of the saffron plant *(Crocus sativus)*, native to Asia Minor, have been dried and ground since Greek and Roman antiquity, and used not only as a spice and coloring agent for food, but also medicinally as an ingredient in pills; as a cleaning and anti-spasmodic agent for the stomach; a nerve tonic and opiate against hysteria and as a relief for nose-bleeds and menstruation.

Saffron, from Mattioli's COMMENTAIRES, *Lyons, 1579.*

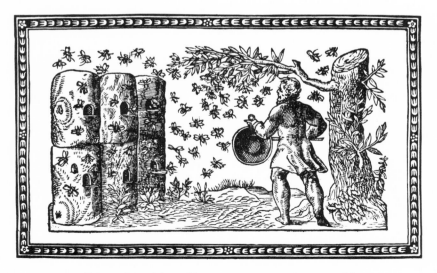

Honey, from Mattioli's COMMENTAIRES, *Lyons, 1579.*

THE CULINARY HERBS

URING THE DARK AGES, the accumulated knowledge of the Persian, Greek and Roman herbalists was nearly lost to humanity. In the 6th century, the Benedictine monks at Monte Cassino in Italy were the only ones who owned a library of herbal manuscripts. They also cultivated the only herb and vegetable garden in all of Europe. These monks copied the gardening and agricultural books in their possession time and again for other monasteries and kept the ancient science of the medicinal and nutritional values of plants alive. In later years it became a rule in every monastery that at least one of the monks acquire a thorough knowledge of plants, their use and cultivation. Finally, it took the invention of printing in the 15th century to popularize this knowledge throughout western Europe and England.

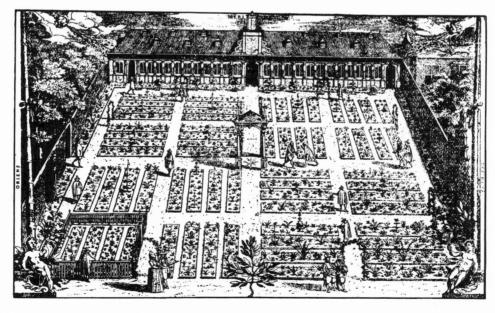

The Botanical Garden at Leiden, by J. C. Woudamus, Holland, 1610.

121

Basil, from Peter Schöffer's HORTUS SANITATIS, *Mainz, 1485.*

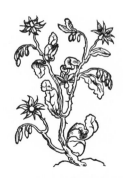

Borage, from Peter Schöffer's HORTUS SANITATIS, *Mainz, 1485.*

SWEET BASIL *(Ocimum basilicum)*, a member of the mint family, native to tropical Asia, Africa and the Pacific Islands, was the most sacred plant in the Hindu gardens of India, worshipped by all members of the family. Its name is derived from the Greek *basilicos* — royal. Sweet basil has been used since pre-Christian times as a cooking herb.

BORAGE *(Borago officinalis)* is a garden herb native to Europe and North Africa. Its name is derived from the Arabic *abu rashsh* — father of sweat, because it was used in antiquity as a sudoriforic. In medieval times, borage leaves were a popular salad green, and wine spiked with borage was considered a remedy for melancholy.

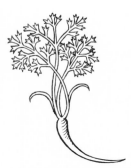

Carrot, from Jacob Meydenbach's ORTUS SANITATIS, *Mainz, 1491.*

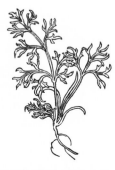

Dill, from Peter Schöffer's HORTUS SANITATIS, *Mainz, 1485.*

CARROT *(Daucus carota)* is a member of the celery family of Eurasian origin. In ancient Greece it was called *Philon*, from the Greek *philo* — loving. Its root was served as a vegetable before amatory affairs because it was believed to possess the power of exciting the passions. It was also believed that raw carrots improve the eyesight.

DILL *(Anethum graveolens)*, an herb of European origin, is believed to be the anise of the Scriptures. Dill seeds have been used since antiquity in cookery, and for flavoring salads and pickles. In medieval times dill was considered a protection against the spell of witches, and when steeped in wine, a potent aphrodisiac and love philtre.

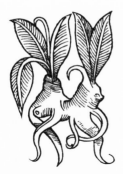

Elecampe, from Crescentius' IN COMMODU
RURALIUM, *Drach, Speyer, 1490.*

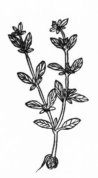

Marjoram, from Peter Schöffer's HORTUS SANITATIS,
Mainz, 1485.

ELECAMPE or **SCABWORT** *(Inula hele-nium)* is a large herb of European and North Asian origin. Its root was used in ancient Rome as a vegetable. In medieval times sweetmeat was made by adding to the ground roots, eggs, salt, sugar, saffron and spices. This herb was also considered an excellent remedy for pulmonary diseases.

MARJORAM *(Origanum vulgare)*, native to southern Europe, has been used since Roman times to give spice and flavor to meats and sauces. Before hop beer was invented, marjoram was used in the brewing of beer and ale. In medieval times, marjoram was considered a powerful charm against witchcraft and marjoram wine a potent antiseptic.

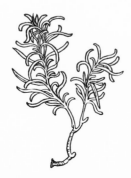

Rosemary, from Peter Schöffer's HORTUS SANITATIS,
Mainz, 1485.

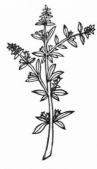

Savory, from Steffen Arndes' HORTUS SANITATIS, *Luebeck, 1492.*

ROSEMARY *(Rosmarinus officinalis)*, native to the Mediterranean region, an herb with a pungent, bitterish taste has been used since early times as a flavoring for fish and sauces. In medieval times a *posset* made from hot, curdled milk and ale, honey and rosemary was considered a great comforter for the heart and a nerve tonic.

SAVORY *(Satureia hortensis)*, an herb of the mint family with a peppery flavor, native to southern Europe, has been used since early antiquity as a salad green and for seasoning poultry. Steeped in wine, it was considered a potent stomach tonic and a remedy for complaints of the liver and the lungs. Powdered, it was used as a flea repellent.

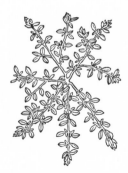

Thyme, from Peter Schöffer's HORTUS SANITATIS, *Mainz, 1485.*

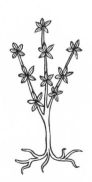

Woodruff, from Steffen Arndes' HORTUS SANITATIS, *Luebeck, 1492.*

WILD THYME (*Thymus serpyllum*) is a creeping shrub of the mint family, native to Europe. Its pungent, lemon-scented, dried tops and leaves have been used since ancient times as a culinary seasoning for soups and meat sauces. In medieval days, thyme mixed with honey was considered a potent remedy for pulmonary diseases.

SWEET WOODRUFF or **WALDMEISTER** (*Asperula odorata*), a small sweet-scented herb of Mediterranean origin, has been used since the early pre-Christian era for flavoring wine. The delicious German *Maitrank*, or Maybowle, made by steeping sprigs of woodruff in Rhine wine, strawberries and sugar, was a blood purifier in medieval times.

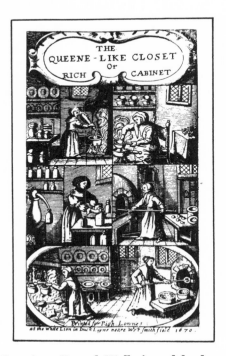

Title Page from Hannah Wolley's cook book, QUEENE-LIKE CLOSET, *London, 1670.*

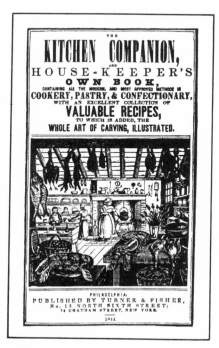

Title Page from Turner & Fisher's KITCHEN COMPANION, *Philadelphia, 1844.*

ILLUSTRATIONS

INDEX